ALZHEIMER'S ESSENTIALS

Practical Skills for Families & Caregivers

Second Edition

BRETTEN C. GORDEAU &
JEFFREY HILLIER PhD

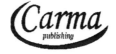
Carma
publishing

Published by Carma Publishing LLC, Delray Beach, Florida, USA

Orders may be placed through the website www.carmapubs.com

© 2007 with the authors

Second Edition May 2007
First Edition July 2005
Updated February 2006

ISBN: 978-0-9769581-7-8
       0-9769581-7-1

The information contained in this publication is believed to be correct at the time of going to press. Neither the authors nor the publisher assume any responsibility for any errors or omissions herein contained. Opinions expressed in the book are those of the authors and are not necessarily held by the publisher. While this book discusses some legal, financial and medical matters, nothing published in this book should be considered legal, financial or medical advice. Readers must always consult a physician, attorney, accountant or other professionals who can assist them concerning matters related to the topic of this book.

Printed in the United States of America

Table of Contents

Acknowledgments

In writing this book, we have compiled information from many sources. We have read avidly; we have had many conversations with experts, patients, and caregivers; and we have the benefit of our own professional and life experiences. We want to thank all of you who have enhanced our knowledge of this terrible disease, whether you were aware of your involvement or not. In particular, we wish to thank Najeeb Qadi MD and Sandra Tam MSc for their chapter on the scientific and medical basis of Alzheimer's disease and to Dr. Howard Feldman, for his guidance in preparing their chapter. We are grateful to Dr. Rachelle Doody for editing and updating Chapter 6 – Therapies. We thank Barbara Caras for helping to make the book what it has become.

This book is dedicated to
all the caregivers who give so much
to care for those who are unable to care for themselves

Foreword

Somewhere lost in the statistics about Alzheimer's disease, are the caregivers. With approximately five million people currently afflicted with Alzheimer's disease in the US, there are 10 to 15 million more people impacted directly by Alzheimer's. These people are caregivers. While much can be found in the literature regarding patients with Alzheimer's disease, very little is written about, studied or provided for the caregivers.

Caregivers are comprised of spouses, family members, friends and professionals. They bear the brunt of this disease, and they are the ones that endure the long nights and periods of loneliness, while they look after their patients. They are the ones in great need of information to help them through the arduous task of caregiving.

Caregiving is as much an art as a science and much is learned from experience. The Alzheimer's Association and support groups can help share some of this experience, and I strongly encourage the caregivers I come into contact with to take advantage of this help.

This handbook is an additional, essential source that can be used both as a guide and as a reference. It is based on the vast experiences of its authors, as well as of those they have come in contact with. I applaud the authors for putting together this valuable book. It is much-needed and provides the information and help for caregivers of all types.

Patrick Gillette M.D.
Director, Memory and Mood Disorder Clinic of So, Oregon

Preface

Since we first published Alzheimer's Essentials in 2005 so many new clinical and research developments have given us a greater insight into the underlying causes, diagnosis and treatment that even though we updated the book in February 2006 we have found it necessary to produce this Second Edition in 2007 to keep it in line with current medical and scientific thinking. While progress is being made in understanding the underlying causes of Alzheimer's and diagnostic skills are being enhanced and more than twenty compounds are in clinical trial in the US, no new medications have been approved since Alzheimer's Essentials was first published. We look forward to the day when we can provide details of medications or other therapies that can reverse the symptoms or even cure this terrible disease.

We are asked frequently why we do not include information about drugs in clinical trials and other advances in this book. The answer is that we have seen so many potential advances and novel medications fail in clinical trials and other tests and we have no way of predicting what may or may not be successful in the future we prefer not to take your time reading about what probably will not happen. We do not want to give hope where there is very little. You can expect that roughly 90% or more of the new drugs in clinical trial will not make it to market either because they do not work, or because the side effects are unacceptable or some other reason. Our hope is that the one or two that do make it to market will make significant improvements in the quality of life for the Alzheimer's patient.

The prevalence of Alzheimer's disease is increasing and the number of families impacted by the disease is rising accordingly. The financial burden associated with the treatment and care of Alzheimer's patients makes it one of the most expensive diseases in the world. The chances are that you know someone with Alzheimer's and so you have picked up this book because you are curious about Alzheimer's disease or dementia. You suspect that you may soon become a caregiver, or a family member or friend may be showing some signs and you just want to know what to expect from this dreadful disease. We have written this little book for you. It provides good information, in an easy to read format, to everyone who wants to know more about what to expect from someone living with Alzheimer's. Having said that, the book is not for the patient, but for you as the caregiver, family member, or friend. The person afflicted with a cognitive disorder such as Alzheimer's should be under the care and treatment of their doctor, so we do not offer any medical advice, but provide the essential information that you will need to prepare yourself for your role as a caregiver. This book is for you because it is your life that will be altered significantly by taking on the role of caregiver to the person living with Alzheimer's.

There is No Known Cure
As a starting point, we should dispel any notion that the person affected is going to get better. As of the writing of this book in 2007, Alzheimer's disease is considered to be incurable and patients will die, on average, 8 years after diagnosis, although they may live as much as 20 years or more after first finding out that they have the disease. In the interim period, they will decline cognitively, grow more confused, remember less and less, and will lose their ability to communicate and care for themselves. While there are treatments that may slow the progression of the disease, death is the end result, often from another sickness such as pneumonia. Patients will decline progressively and even though they may have moments of lucidity in the later stages, do not think there is hope for a recovery. There is not, but you can learn to enjoy the moments of lucidity and the time you spend together.

Approximately 75% of patients end up in a health care facility 5 years from diagnosis and this is the kind of situation for which you have to plan. In this book, we provide you with enough information to make you aware of the crucial decisions you may have to make to care for the person with Alzheimer's and to manage your own life. The role of the caregiver is not an easy one, but with good planning and armed with knowledge, we believe that your life can be made a little easier and, perhaps, even rewarding.

You, the caregiver, should expect that the person with Alzheimer's will be totally dependent on you eventually and, for this reason, your role as the caregiver is integral to the development of any plan of care for the patient. Therefore, we want to help you to understand what you should expect in your new role.

Myths

The cause of Alzheimer's disease remains virtually unknown, with the exception of the ~25% of familial genetic cases. While research continues to explore the potential causes of Alzheimer's, a few myths that are unproven by scientific evidence have become popular to explain the cause of the disease. Until scientific evidence proves otherwise, these explanations should be considered nothing more than folklore.

o   The disease is caused by components found in soda cans, cooking utensils, and deodorants.
o   The disease is caused by a viral or bacterial infection.
o   Alzheimer's is the natural progress of aging.
o   Alzheimer's is curable.
o   We know how Alzheimer's can be prevented.
o   Gingko biloba, primrose oil, and other supplements such as lecithin, DHEA (dehydroepiandrosterone – a naturally occurring steroid hormone), acetyl-l-carnitine, and ginseng are effective treatments.

Be wary of any claims made on the Internet, in magazines, or late-night infomercials that claim to have a cure for memory loss; these agents are inherently snake oil. There is no cure. There is no known cause. What you *can* have faith in is that there are modestly effective treatments that can be prescribed by your doctor and these may slow the progression of Alzheimer's.

We have kept this book short by design. We want you to get the essential information in an easy-to-read format. We have provided a Glossary to help with the words that may be unfamiliar to you, and we have provided some Internet and literature references to help you to follow up and learn more. We update the information in this book on a regular basis so that you will always have the most recent information as new ideas become known to us and as the research and medical communities make progress. The latest update is this Second Edition published in May 2007.

We welcome your feedback and suggestions and you can contact us easily from the www.carmapubs.com website or by emailing us at publisher@carmapubs.com.

About the Authors

Bretten C. Gordeau is a memory impairment specialist who has worked directly with hundreds of Alzheimer's and memory impaired patients, families and caregivers in long term care and day care settings. He has provided educational programs on Alzheimer's disease practice to more than 400 clinicians. He has spent the past ten years working within neurology, neurosurgery research and publishing as well as being appointed to state advisory and county committees and advocating on a government level for those living with memory impairments within California. He holds seats on various boards of directors for neurodegenerative disorders. Mr. Gordeau is also a long distance caregiver for his father who is living with a neurodegenerative brain impairment and has had two other family members affected by a dementia. He attended Harvard and Cambridge Universities and completed his surgical science studies at the University of Miami Medical School Campus.

Jeffrey Hillier received his PhD in neuropharmacology from the University of Bath, England. He has held senior management positions in several of the world's leading publishing companies and is a founder of Carma Publishing. He has an intense interest in the biology and medicine of neurological disorders and the ways in which patients and caregivers are impacted.

.

Other books for Families & Caregivers

Bipolar Essentials

Other books on Alzheimer's Disease and Dementia

Alzheimer's Dementia edited by Rachelle S Doody MD PhD

Parkinson's Dementia edited by Clive Ballard MD

Huntington's Dementia edited by Blair Leavitt MD

Other Dementias edited by David Geldmacher MD

To order any of these books or for an update on all books
from Carma Publishing visit
www.carmapubs.com

1. An Introduction to Dementia

First Signs

The first signs of "something being wrong" will be noticed by the individual themselves or by a spouse, family member, or friend. Symptoms should not be ignored, especially if the person is older. If you notice problems with remembering things or significant changes in mental functions (such as increased forgetfulness, confusion, or personality changes), this could indicate dementia and it is time to discuss the symptoms with your spouse, family members, or friends and to seek the advice of a primary care practitioner so that a diagnosis for the problems can be provided. If the loss of memory gets worse over time, there is reason to be concerned and the patient should visit their doctor for a checkup.

Memory loss and forgetfulness are a part of the normal aging process so there may be nothing to be concerned about and becoming forgetful does not necessarily mean that the person has dementia or Alzheimer's disease. As a rule of thumb, those with age-related memory loss are often able to recall eventually what they had forgotten, whereas the memory loss due to Alzheimer's is more severe. People with Alzheimer's, in the long term, are more likely to forget people and entire experiences rather than just parts of them, and are rarely able to recall the experience at all.

If you have concerns about memory loss in a family member or friend and if you believe the answer is "yes" to any of the following questions, it is time for you to talk to the person affected and work with them to schedule a visit to their doctor for a checkup:

- o   Are they forgetting things much more frequently than they used to?
- o   Are they forgetting things they have done many times in the past?
- o   Is memory loss affecting their daily living?

- o Do people tell them they are repeating themselves during the same conversation?
- o Are they having trouble making choices?
- o Are they having trouble paying bills and handling their financial affairs?
- o Are they finding that they cannot keep track of what they are doing?
- o Are they having trouble learning new things?

Only health care professionals have the knowledge and experience to diagnose Alzheimer's and other forms of dementia. If a form of dementia is diagnosed, the sooner treatment is started, the better. Plans must be made to take care of the person who may be diagnosed with a dementia and to take care of your own life as the caregiver.

Alzheimer's is generally considered to be the most common form of dementia, although there is some evidence that frontotemporal dementia (FTD) is just as common. This latter form of dementia does not occur with a memory loss as obvious as that due to Alzheimer's, however.

If the individual is diagnosed with Alzheimer's, they may be able to maximize their quality of life by receiving an early diagnosis. An early diagnosis allows more time to plan for the future and an opportunity to make decisions concerning care, living and financial arrangements, and legal and other important issues. Also, the sooner the person diagnosed receives therapy and enrolls in social model day care, even though there is no cure, the more the progressive deterioration in cognitive function and memory loss seen in Alzheimer's can be delayed. The longer the person is able to take care of themselves to some degree, the better the situation will be for the caregiver and the immediate costs for the person affected, the caregiver, and society are reduced. The pharmacoeconomic benefits (cost benefits of using prescription therapies) of drug therapy will be discussed later in this book.

In recent times, physicians have altered their view of memory loss such that a certain degree of memory loss may indicate to them that some disease process is affecting the brain. People complaining of memory loss should expect to be tested for cognitive function by their doctor so that a diagnosis can be made. The outcome of these tests will show the severity of memory loss and decline in cognitive function, and will lead to a diagnosis. The diagnosis may be that the memory loss is typical of old age and no further action other than follow-up visits is necessary. If the tests indicate more severe problems, a diagnosis of mild cognitive impairment (MCI) (sometimes also called CIND – Cognitive Impairment, Not Dementia) or a form of dementia may be applied. Some doctors do not recognize MCI as a separate disease classification but consider the symptoms as early Alzheimer's disease. For the purposes of this discussion we will use the term MCI.

Although Alzheimer's is characterized by a steady deterioration and other forms of cognitive impairment may come and go, it can be challenging to differentiate between minor memory lapses and significant memory loss.

So What is Mild Cognitive Impairment?
Individuals with MCI show greater memory impairment on formal memory tests when compared with normal aging patients, but lack the cognitive deficits of patients with Alzheimer's disease. So, the MCI patient may forget names, where they put things, and they may have trouble remembering the flow of a conversation, but they are able to perform all their usual functions without the assistance of others. The MCI patient will be able to compensate for their memory loss by using tools such as writing notes, using calendars, or pocket computers or PDAs.

So, for now, a diagnosis of MCI should be a relief, as the patient can be expected to continue to function independently. However, obtaining a diagnosis is important so that further visits to their doctor can be scheduled and so that their symptoms can be monitored and any further deterioration recognized immediately and medication started if their doctor so decides.

Memory complaints in the elderly are associated with a higher risk of dementia development. Most commonly, the type of dementia that patients with MCI are at risk to develop is Alzheimer's, though other dementias (such as vascular dementia or FTD) may develop as well. However, some people diagnosed with MCI never develop a dementia at all. Unfortunately, there is no way to predict which patients diagnosed with MCI will go on to develop a dementia. From the caregiver's viewpoint, you should be aware that a diagnosis of MCI means that the person diagnosed has an increased risk of developing a dementia and you should already start to make plans in the event that the dementia does develop. You should be keeping a close eye on them, looking for signs of the condition worsening, and make sure that follow-up visits to the doctor take place as scheduled.

While there is currently no specific treatment for MCI, as new medications for Alzheimer's are developed in the future, these are likely to be tried on patients with MCI as well. If data from such trials indicate a beneficial effect in slowing cognitive decline, the importance of recognizing MCI and identifying it early will increase. Some physicians may choose to use Alzheimer's therapies when treating MCI, as some studies have shown that early intervention may help to reduce the rate of cognitive decline.

And What is Dementia?
Dementia is a broad term used to indicate degenerative brain disease and refers to a group of symptoms that are the result of the deterioration of mental functioning such that normal independent functions like thinking, remembering, reasoning, and judgment are impossible and the symptoms are severe enough to hinder everyday activities (activities of daily living – ADLs) and social relationships. Alzheimer's disease is one of many kinds of dementia and is probably the most common. Examples of some of the more prevalent symptoms of dementia can be found in Chapter 4.

What is Alzheimer's Disease?
It is named after Dr. Alois Alzheimer who, in 1906, discovered the disease at autopsy of a 57-year-old woman. Alzheimer found some distinctive changes in the woman's brain distinguished by abnormal clumps now known as amyloid or neuritic plaques, and abnormal tangled bundles of nerve fibers now known as neurofibrillary tangles. Alzheimer's disease is a progressive, degenerative brain disease characterized by memory impairment and accompanied by a gradual decline in the patient's ability to perform ADLs, adverse

changes in behavior and personality, and a decline in cognitive functions such as language and executive functioning. Alzheimer's is the leading cause of dementia in people over the age of 65, with an average age at onset of 72.8 years. The symptoms of Alzheimer's become more severe with time as the brain tissue progressively degenerates, causing a reduction in brain size as the neurons die. Over an average of 8 years, Alzheimer's shuts down the functions of the brain, beginning with immediate and short-term memory, then shifting to language and basic thinking skills, bladder and bowel incontinence, and finally impairing mobility and basic life functions like swallowing and breathing. For those who do not die of an unrelated condition in the interim, such as pneumonia, Alzheimer's is always fatal. The average survival time for a person over 65 is 8.3 years after diagnosis, whereas a 90-year-old person's average survival is just 3.4 years.

Some statistical information is useful to put Alzheimer's into a societal context. Each year, in the Unites States, about 100,000 people die from Alzheimer's and approximately 360,000 new cases are diagnosed. It is estimated that at least 5 million people in the U.S. suffer from the disease and some sources project the number to rise to 14 million or more by 2050. Worldwide, the estimated prevalence of the disease in 2005 was 29.3 million people with Alzheimer's and dementia and it is estimated that about 10% - 12% of all individuals will suffer some form of dementia. Studies show that people experience symptoms from 3.5–5.5 years before receiving a diagnosis. An estimated 42% of all people 85 and older have symptoms of Alzheimer's and 19% of people between ages 75 and 84 are affected. Roughly 2% in the 65 to 74 age group are expected to develop Alzheimer's disease. As America's population grows older, the number of people with Alzheimer's will increase and could double every 20 years.

Start a Family Medical History. Once a diagnosis for Alzheimer's disease has been made, you should inform all the family members and start a family medical history that includes the Alzheimer's diagnosis. The family history may be useful for family members to prepare for their own futures with or without the possibility of having Alzheimer's.

Who is at Risk for Alzheimer's Disease?
The leading risk factors for developing Alzheimer's disease are generally considered to be the following:

Age — No one is immune to Alzheimer's and there is no known preventive measure. The cause is still not known, but risk increases dramatically with age. It is almost unheard of in people aged 20–39 and very uncommon (about 1 in 2,500) for people aged 40–59. In the 60s, however, the odds begin to get more worrisome. It is estimated that the following age groups have Alzheimer's or a closely related dementia:

- o 1% of 65 year olds
- o 2% of 68 year olds
- o 3% of 70 year olds
- o 6% of 73 year olds
- o 9% of 75 year olds
- o 13% of 77 year olds

And so on. The risk accelerates with age to the point where dementia affects nearly half of those 85 and over. Because Alzheimer's can strike people in their 40s and 50s, this early-onset form of the disease presents unique planning issues for the individual and caregiver. Because of their longer life span, women are at higher risk than men for cognitive impairment.

Genetic factors — The causes of dementing diseases are unknown although ongoing research studies have found links between genetic mutations and Alzheimer's disease (see Chapter 9). What we do know is that about 25% of Alzheimer's cases are familial i.e. two or more persons in a family have Alzheimer's disease. Less than 2% are diagnosed as early-onset (onset before age 65) familial Alzheimer's disease, with approximately 23% diagnosed as late-onset (after age 65) familial Alzheimer's disease. The remaining 75% of the Alzheimer's population has unknown causes for their disease and of this larger group the vast majority will suffer late-onset Alzheimer's disease.

Anyone who has a parent, sibling or offspring with Alzheimer's is approximately 2.5 times more likely to develop Alzheimer's than someone who does not have a close relative with the disease. This means that if you have a parent, sibling or offspring with Alzheimer's disease you have a 20 – 25% chance of also developing Alzheimer's.

The greatest risk factor for developing Alzheimer's or dementia is age, but certain other lifestyle factors have been associated with a higher incidence of Alzheimer's:

Cardiovascular diseases — Studies have shown that people at risk for heart disease (such as people with high blood pressure and high cholesterol) are at a higher risk for developing dementia than people without these risk factors. Those who have been diagnosed with hypertension are 24% more likely to develop dementia and those with high cholesterol were 42% more likely to develop dementia.

Smoking — According to a paper published in the medical journal *Neurology*, a study conducted over a 41-year period revealed that of 9,000 people examined in Northern California, those who were smokers had a 26% higher risk of developing dementia.

Diabetes — Individuals with diabetes are 46% more likely to develop dementia.

Stress — There are indications that stress hormones play a role in the development of mild cognitive impairment (MCI) and Alzheimer's disease. Animal studies have shown that stress hormones exacerbate the formation of brain lesions associated with Alzheimer's disease. It has been postulated that people susceptible to stress may be at a higher risk for developing Alzheimer's.

Multiple factors — With a combination of these risk factors (hypertension, high cholesterol, diabetes, and smoking) and the average risk factor being equal to 27%, increased risk jumps to a 237% chance of developing dementia if you have all four risk factors compared to those without these factors.

Stroke — The results of a study published in the journal *Stroke* suggest that patients who have suffered a stroke have twice the risk of dementia compared with healthy individuals.

Obesity — A U.S. study has indicated that people who are obese in their 40s have a 74% greater likelihood of developing dementia when compared to people of "normal" weight and people who are overweight have a 35% greater chance of developing dementia. Overweight or obesity was measured by the body mass index (BMI) method. For those of you concerned about your weight, you can calculate BMI by dividing your weight in kilograms (1 kilogram = 2.205 pounds) by the square of your height in meters (1 meter = 3.3 feet). If the answer is greater than 25, you are overweight. If it is greater than 30, you are obese. Obese women seem to be at greater risk, having a 200% greater chance of developing dementia than women of normal weight, whereas obese men had a 30% greater risk. A Swedish study has shown that the higher a woman's BMI, the greater the chance they would experience brain tissue loss, one of the first signs of a developing dementia.

Depression — Many patients with depression also complain about loss of memory.

Education — It has been suggested that high levels of education may help to preserve brain function because of the increased number of brain connections. Also, keeping the brain active as it ages has been suggested as being important in maintaining brain function and delaying the onset of Alzheimer's symptoms. There are many books, games and classes focusing on memory improvement and keeping the brain active as a way to improve memory as we get older. The evidence seems to be that these activities help and we certainly encourage our readers to consider these activities if they are noticing memory problems.

Nutrition — The potential effect of diet and nutrition on dementia and cognitive impairment is a subject of increasing scientific interest. In particular, there are studies that have produced evidence that nutrients such as vitamins, trace elements and lipids can affect the risk of cognitive decline especially in the frail and elderly population. Since some of the studies have produced conflicting results, there is no clear cut answer on what nutrients help and what nutrients harm. However, on the negative side, high intake of saturated and trans-unsaturated fats has been associated with an increased risk of Alzheimer's disease. On the positive side, the good fats, polyunsaturated and monounsaturated have been associated with protection against cognitive decline in the elderly.

Vitamins, especially vitamins B9 and B12 have also been associated with a protective role in cognitive decline and dementia.

Studies in animals and humans indicate that people with low levels of folate in their blood are at higher risk to develop Alzheimer's disease. Folate or folic acid is a constituent of a healthy diet and is found in leafy green vegetables, asparagus, broccoli, liver, and many types of beans and peas, as well as fruits such as oranges and bananas, as well as being a constituent of fortified bread.

A recent study indicated that drinking fruit and vegetable juices regularly may reduce the risk of developing Alzheimer's disease. The researchers found the risk of Alzheimer's developing was 76% lower for those who drank juice more than three times a week, compared with those who drank it less than once a week. The juices are thought to neutralize the damaging effects of free radicals in the brain.

In yet another study researchers found that people who eat a "Mediterranean" diet rich in fruits, vegetables, olive oil, legumes, cereals and fish have a lower risk of developing Alzheimer's disease,

Consult with your doctor before changing your diet or taking supplements such as vitamin pills.

Other factors — Several studies have suggested that certain measurements of atrophy (shrinkage) or decreased metabolism on images of the brain (PET – positron emission tomography or MRI – magnetic resonance imaging scans) increase the chances of developing dementia in the future.

Many variables contribute to memory loss and cognitive dysfunction, such as environment, trauma, genetics, and even drug interactions or overmedication. According to various Alzheimer's resources, those individuals who are proactive about addressing their health issues, who manage their risk factors and who exercise regularly have less chance statistically of developing a dementia.

Can we Predict who will get Alzheimer's Disease?

Even though more and more is known about MCI and Alzheimer's disease and researchers and physicians are constantly modifying how they diagnose and treat these diseases, there has not been a reliable predictor of who may develop Alzheimer's. However, a new risk analysis tool, developed in Sweden, called the Dementia Risk Score may soon be in clinical use to assess those most at risk such as relatives and family members of those suffering from Alzheimer's disease. Age, education, high systolic blood pressure, obesity, high cholesterol and inactivity are all taken into account in this predictive test in which a high score in mid-life is a predictor of a higher likelihood of developing dementia.

Progression of Alzheimer's Disease

Alzheimer's disease causes a global loss of intellectual abilities that is severe enough to interfere with daily functioning. Initial symptoms are subtle; the person may show signs of personality change, memory loss, poor judgment, have less initiative, be unable to learn new things, have mood swings, or become easily agitated. Gradually, as the disease progresses, the victim develops speech and language problems, movement and coordination difficulties, bowel and bladder incontinence, total confusion and disorientation, and will ultimately rely completely on a caregiver for daily functioning. Although the victim may appear completely healthy in the early stages of Alzheimer's, the disease is slowly destroying the brain cells. This hidden process damages the brain in several ways:

- o Patches of brain cells degenerate (neuritic plaques).
- o Nerve endings that transmit messages within the brain become tangled (neurofibrillary tangles).
- o There is a reduction in acetylcholine, an important neurotransmitter in the brain.
- o Spaces in the brain (ventricles, holding ponds for cerebrospinal fluid) become larger and filled with a granular fluid.
- o The size and shape of the brain alters. The cortex appears to shrink and decay.

For those of you interested in the pathophysiology (the functional changes associated with or resulting from the disease) of Alzheimer's, we have provided more information in Chapter 9.

Understandably, as the brain continues to degenerate, there is a comparable loss in mental functioning. Since the brain controls all of our bodily functions, an Alzheimer's victim in the later stages will have difficulty walking, talking, swallowing, controlling bladder and bowel functions, etc. The individual becomes quite frail and prone to infections such as pneumonia.

To complicate the diagnostic procedures further, there are numerous conditions that mimic Alzheimer's. Conditions such as stroke (without multi-infarct dementia), vascular diseases (without vascular dementia), toxins, vitamin (such as B12) and nutritional deficiencies, depression, infections, and mismanagement of medications can all have symptoms that mimic Alzheimer's. For this very reason, it is most important that a thorough examination be done in order to rule out any treatable conditions.

What is the Cost?
Alzheimer's disease is the third most expensive disease in the U.S., costing more than $100 billion a year with an additional $33 billion a year in lost productivity. The cost worldwide was estimated to be $315.4 billion in 2005. About three-quarters of Alzheimer's patients are admitted to some form of long-term care within 5 years of diagnosis and it is the cost of stay at a long-term care facility (including the need for skilled nursing in the last few years of the individual's life) that leads to the high cost of care for the person with Alzheimer's. This can place a large financial burden on the caregiver and family, but long-term care does play a vital role in the well being of both the family and the person with Alzheimer's. When drug therapies are administered that can delay the progression of the disease so that the person with Alzheimer's can be less dependent and can remain at home while enrolled in a social model day care and respite service, then we should see that the cost to the caregiver and immediate family is reduced in the short term. Scientific studies have shown that when acetylcholinesterase inhibitors are given to individuals with Alzheimer's, the time taken

to care for the individual is reduced by between 1 and 2 hours per week, easing the burden of care and potential caregiver burnout.

The comforting part of these numbers is that if you or someone you know is diagnosed with Alzheimer's, you are not alone, and while the disease remains incurable, it seems likely that the research effort into a cure from both the private and public sectors will escalate until a cure is found or much improved medications are discovered that will stop the progression of the disease or even reverse the disease process. Equally important to finding a cure and better medications is the need for an accurate test to diagnose Alzheimer's. Current research into finding biochemical markers (clues in the body) for Alzheimer's is showing promising results, although it will still be several years before any biochemical tests are available for use by physicians. Diagnostic imaging is showing promise as a detection tool to diagnose Alzheimer's and may be available routinely in the clinic in the not too distant future if the insurance companies will cover the cost.

Studies have indicated that Alzheimer's is as costly as treating diabetes and heart disease, and nearly as expensive as treating cancer. According to Alzheimer's Association statistics, the lifetime cost per individual can be as high as $174,000. The cost of treatment to Medicare averages $13,207 per person per year. Metlife, the insurance company, has estimated that the work of unpaid caregivers would be worth $257 billion per year if performed by paid home care workers, and working caregivers who go from full-time to part-time status or leave a job to perform their caregiver responsibilities experience an average lifetime total wealth loss of approximately $659,000.

The cost of treating other sicknesses (comorbid illnesses are very common in the elderly) in individuals with a dementia in a managed-care setting is much higher than the costs for treating non-demented patients. The reason for this is because patients with dementia are less able to participate in their own care and are less able to follow the instructions of their doctor. So, treating the dementia with available medications can prove beneficial for the treatment of the individual's comorbid illnesses.

Alzheimer's is a very expensive illness, not just in terms of economic cost, but also in terms of human cost. This is a family illness. It is not just the patient who is impacted by the disease; Alzheimer's also has tremendous impact on the caregivers' health and lifestyles.

2. Talking to Your Doctor

One of the primary responsibilities of the caregiver is to act as the go-between for the doctor and the patient. The caregiver provides information to the doctor about the patient and assists the patient in following the doctor's orders. You, as the caregiver, are the only advocate for the person with Alzheimer's disease because they are unable to advocate for themselves. In most cases, the best advocates for people with Alzheimer's are those who have known them the longest, probably a spouse or family member.

The diagnosis of Alzheimer's can be very difficult for many primary care practitioners, especially if they work in a community with few older residents. It is not uncommon for Alzheimer's to be diagnosed incorrectly. This makes it even more important that you communicate effectively with the doctor to obtain an accurate diagnosis and to make sure that you are informed of all the options for therapy. (We provide information on diagnosis in Chapter 4 and on therapy in Chapter 6.) At the present time, statistics indicate that as many as half of the patients developing Alzheimer's are not diagnosed or are misdiagnosed. Of those that are diagnosed, two-thirds to three-quarters are not treated despite the fact that many studies now show that the progression of Alzheimer's can be slowed with existing medicines.

Health care today is much different than it was 20 years ago. Doctors are busier than ever and they have limited time available, so communicating effectively with the doctor is more important than it ever was. You may wait for an extended amount of time both in the waiting room and exam room, and once you do see the doctor your visit may be no more than 15 minutes. Because time is so limited, it is important that you should be prepared. Communication is the sharpest tool you have available to you and how well you are able to talk with the doctor may affect the care of the person with Alzheimer's. The relationship between doctor and caregiver should be one based on the sharing of information and working together to make the best decisions about the patient's health, resulting in the best care being provided.

Preparing for Your Visit to the Doctor's Office
It is important to involve family members or friends to help you to prepare and to accompany you to the appointment. Involving others may help you to be more accurate and focused, leading to a more productive discussion with the doctor. By having someone visit the doctor with you, they act as another set of ears and can act as a second voice when relaying complicated health information to the family or to each other. It will be helpful to the doctor and to help communication between all the family members if one person, usually the primary caregiver, serves as the main contact and informant. This person should plan on being at all of the appointments with the doctor.

Focusing on the current state of the individual with Alzheimer's disease and their general health condition will help to prevent misunderstandings. Asking questions and focusing on relevant items may encourage the doctor to take more time with you. Do not make the doctor guess or come to conclusions; be precise and clear. The more information you share, the better the doctor will be able to figure out the best diagnosis and treatment options.

The best way to make the most of the limited time you will have with the doctor is to come to your appointment prepared. Make your lists of questions and prepare the information you will give to the doctor with a friend or family member a few days before the appointment. Include the following:

o   Gather both over-the-counter (aspirin, vitamins, etc.) and prescription medications and make a list of the names, monthly quantity, dosing instructions, and dosage with the name and phone number of the pharmacy where the medications were purchased. Also, include the name of the doctor if different to the one you will be visiting.

o   Make a list of symptoms, such as "mother is getting lost going to the store, my husband can't understand how to balance the check book, my brother is not able to remember what I've just said to him," etc. It is also important to write how often these examples occur.

o List any previous health problems (including past surgeries) and any relevant or similar symptoms or diagnoses in family members.

o Take along the patient's weight history. A loss of weight may be a sign of Alzheimer's disease (See Chapter 4) and it is important for your doctor to know of any loss of weight especially if there is no apparent cause.

o Make note of any increases in falls and loss of balance as falling is seen as a symptom in the progression of Alzheimer's disease.

The next step is to think about why you are going to see the doctor and how to use the time effectively. Focus on the following to best communicate your needs and those of your loved one:

o The appointment is to discuss the important issues you are about to face, such as your loved one's independence, needs, treatments, and if they are still driving, how to establish that they cannot drive any longer.

o The appointment is not to discuss your own complaints.

o Focus on the future. If this is early diagnosis, focus on the best treatment options, activities, and ways to help your loved one prepare. If in the mild stages, find out what to expect for the next 5–10 years and treatment options. If they are in the middle stages of the illness, request a roadmap for the next 5 years and the treatment options.

At the Doctor's Office

A doctor who is well versed in the treatment and diagnosis of dementias will ask you specific questions about the person and will be able to discuss disease care. They can also refer you to the resources you need, such as a day care or respite care facility.

The doctor may do the following:

o Ask about the person's common ADLs, such as getting dressed, eating, picking out clothes, or taking medication.

o Explain about diagnostic tests, such as a Mini Mental State

Exam (MMSE), MRI, or PET and that he will diagnose in the next appointment after testing.

o   Perform an MMSE and give a diagnosis and explain what to expect in the future.
o   Schedule the next visit and let you know how often you should come back.

If you do not understand what the doctor is telling you or they are using medical jargon or words that you do not understand, ask them to explain it again. Using different (layperson's) words or drawing or showing you an illustration can help you to understand. Make sure to bring up anything that you want to discuss that the doctor may not have mentioned or discussed. Do not leave the office without understanding everything the doctor told you. Make sure you tell the doctor everything that you know about the individual's general health, including all symptoms and problems.

Doctors often are so focused on their patient load or the time allotted to each patient that they can be impatient or rushed and they may forget to talk about the disease, further diagnostic testing, or treatment options. If a misunderstanding arises during your appointment, promptly discuss it with the doctor.

Do not be afraid to ask specific questions. These questions are important for you to ask and to have answered, and do not worry if you get home and realize that you have forgotten to ask some of your questions. Make another list and either fax or e-mail the questions with a request for an answer, call the doctor, or take them on your next visit. Here are some questions that you should ask if the doctor is suspecting a dementia:

o   What does the diagnosis mean? Can you explain it in a way that I will understand?
o   Should we seek a specialist?
o   How many patients do you treat with dementia or Alzheimer's disease?
o   What medications are available for memory loss or for behavior changes?
o   What are the risks and benefits of the medication?

- Are there any treatments that work together or in conjunction with one another?
- What are the side effects?
- How long will my loved one take this medicine?
- Should we consider participating in a drug trial?
- What are the risks and benefits?
- Under what circumstances should we call your office?
- What can we expect in the near future and over time?
- Do you have any written material on this disease? If not, who does?
- Are there any organizations or community services that can help?
- Is there anything that we can change at home to make things easier or safer?
- Is there anything else we should know?

When you are concluding your visit, do not forget to ask for referrals or recommendations for community support that can help you to prepare for the daily challenges of caregiving. As well, review what you have just learned with your friend or family member who has accompanied you to the visit.

After the Visit to the Doctor's Office
It is a good idea to make a diary of day-to-day activities and any changes that occur with the person affected, as this will be helpful for subsequent visits:

- Changes in symptoms (memory, mood, behavior) — When they started, frequency, time of day.
- How the prescribed treatments are working — What has improved; what has worsened?
- Any possible changes in mood, behavior, or activity since the start of new medications.
- Make notes about their general health, such as fatigue, infrequent bowel movements, problems with incontinence, headaches, irritability, listlessness, etc.
- As the caregiver, you should also list what is happening with your mental and physical health.
- And list any questions about additional help that you may need.

The person with Alzheimer's disease creates many challenges for the caregiver and for the clinicians who treat them. Working together as a team will help to create a supportive environment that can provide a foundation for adequate and effective care, creating a better quality of life for the person living with Alzheimer's.

3. Diagnosis and Prognosis

The diagnosis of dementia can be difficult. Deciding between normal aging, MCI, and dementia, and deciding between the different kinds of dementia (a listing of the most common forms of dementia is provided at the end of this chapter), is a challenge for many primary care physicians. However, the importance of receiving an early and accurate diagnosis cannot be overstated, so it is important to get it right. The diagnostic tests that are currently available should enable the physician to make an accurate diagnosis.

Once the decision has been made to seek a diagnosis from a primary care practitioner, geriatrician, specialty neurologist, or a primary care physician with dementia treatment experience, it is helpful for you to understand the elements of the diagnostic process and the different stages of Alzheimer's disease that might be diagnosed. An understanding of the process and the symptoms is important for the person showing possible signs of Alzheimer's and for potential caregivers, since the diagnosis of Alzheimer's continues to be missed in clinical practice. If you are concerned that something might have been missed, you should discuss your concerns with the doctor and understand the rationale for the diagnosis. If you remain concerned, seek a second opinion. Do not be afraid that you will offend your doctor by seeking a second opinion. An accurate and early diagnosis is important in order to initiate treatment and to help extend quality of life.

The diagnosis of Alzheimer's is usually considered in three phases: mild, moderate, and severe although as many as seven stages have been defined (see http://alz.org/AboutAD/Stages.asp for more detail). In mild and moderate cases, more than half are not correctly diagnosed and of those that are diagnosed, only two-thirds to three-quarters are treated despite the availability of drugs that are useful in delaying the progression of the disease. We have already seen the huge cost of Alzheimer's in the U.S. and any postponement of the progression of the disease or delay in the onset of symptoms has large potential cost benefits to you as the caregiver and to American society in general, let alone the social benefits you will enjoy by looking after an individual who is more able to take care of themselves and interact with others.

The sooner an accurate diagnosis is made, the easier it will be to manage symptoms and plan for the future.

Before we proceed with a discussion of the diagnosis, we want to remind you that the prognosis for a person with Alzheimer's is not good. A person with Alzheimer's can generally expect to live about 8 years from the time of diagnosis, although many factors, including the person's overall health, cause life expectancy to vary and patients may live for 20 or more years after diagnosis.

There have been astounding advances in Alzheimer's research in recent years, leading many researchers to be hopeful that effective treatments will become available over the next 5–15 years. Several potential breakthrough drugs are already in human trials, but it is unlikely that anyone already diagnosed with Alzheimer's will benefit from drugs now in the research phase. The next generation of Alzheimer's patients may have a better prognosis. This does not mean that you should give up, however. As you read through this book, you will find helpful tips that you can apply to make your time easier and enjoy the person's company for as long as possible.

There are a few drugs available right now that are sometimes helpful in treating the symptoms of Alzheimer's for a limited time (see Chapter 6). Patients and caregivers should consult a doctor about whether the available drugs might be suited to them and make sure that the doctor informs them of all available therapies, including combination therapies. Untreated, the symptoms of Alzheimer's may progress more quickly. The drugs that are currently available, when effective, slow down the progression and relieve some of the symptoms of Alzheimer's.

Current research is showing very promising progress in the development of diagnostic tests for Alzheimer's. Reliable tests should lead to earlier diagnoses as well as more accurate diagnoses. It is generally believed that if Alzheimer's is discovered early enough in the patient, the chances of effectively treating the disease are enhanced. One recent study using brain scans showed that changes in brain structure could be identified an average of four years before a diagnosis of mild cognitive impairment could be made. If these results can be confirmed there is a possibility that at least those at high risk can be screened and preventive strategies tried.

The Family's Role in Diagnosis

In the first (mild) stages of diagnosis, the symptoms do not interfere dramatically with everyday life. For this reason, the symptoms of Alzheimer's disease are often mistaken as a normal part of growing older. It is important, therefore, that the family stays vigilant and looks for the symptoms worsening over time — a sign that Alzheimer's or other dementia may be the cause.

While some individuals may recognize the symptoms themselves, it is often up to a family member to alert the physician and to make arrangements for a visit to the doctor's office and to accompany the patient to the doctor's appointment. The family member can help provide answers to the doctor's questions, such as:

o   What symptoms have you noticed?
o   When did the symptoms first appear?
o   How have the symptoms changed over time?
o   Does the person suffer from other medical conditions?
o   Is the person taking medications? If so, what?
o   Is there a family history of Alzheimer's?
o   Have you noticed personality changes, such as depression, irritability, mean-spiritedness, weeping, mood swings, etc.?
o   Has there been a devastating event, such as the death of a spouse or close friend? Illness? Surgery? Have you noticed if they have become more distant, fatigued, or uninterested in socializing after the event?

Diagnosing Alzheimer's Disease

The diagnosis of Alzheimer's disease is one of excluding other conditions that may be responsible for producing the symptoms of memory loss, confusion, personality change, etc. There is no specific "test" to determine Alzheimer's; the only definitive diagnosis is given after a postmortem brain autopsy has been performed.

Since there are numerous conditions that mimic the symptoms of Alzheimer's, a thorough evaluation is necessary in order to rule out any condition that may be treatable. A neurologist, memory disorder clinic, or hospital with a specialized geriatric program can do effective evaluations.

Establishing a Cognitive Baseline
One of the first steps for the physician is to create a cognitive baseline. This is to establish the level of cognitive functioning at the time the diagnosis is being made so that at future visits the doctor will have something against which to compare changes in functioning. It is necessary to establish a cognitive baseline that can be used as a benchmark for confirming cognitive decline, evaluating its nature and magnitude, and measuring the effectiveness of therapies. To differentiate Alzheimer's disease from normal aging, assessing cognitive decline over time is the most useful diagnostic procedure. It may be necessary to repeat mental status testing over a 6-to 12-month period to compare the results with the results from the initial tests and draw the appropriate conclusions about any decline in cognitive functioning.

Diagnostic Tests
A typical evaluation of a patient with suspected Alzheimer's disease generally includes the following:

o   Social/medical history.
o   Sensory/motor exams.
o   Depression screening.
o   Medication review.
o   Mental status exams.
o   CT (computed tomography) SCAN or MRI (can show brain atrophy, shrinkage, tumors, strokes).
o   Blood tests, urine tests, vitamin deficiencies (such as B12), thyroid testing.
o   Psychosocial and behavioral testing.

If indicated by specific physical findings, other tests may be included, such as:

- o Lumbar puncture (determines malignancies, infections).
- o PET or SPECT (single photon emission computed tomography) SCAN (allows brain functioning to be evaluated).
- o EEG (electroencephalography) (shows brainwave activity).

There is no one diagnostic test that can detect if a person has Alzheimer's. The diagnosis is made by reviewing a detailed history of the person and the results of several tests, including a complete physical and neurological examination, a psychiatric evaluation, and laboratory tests. The primary care practitioner can often handle the diagnosis, although sometimes a team of physicians may be employed. The diagnostic tests usually take more than one day and may involve going to several locations or to a specialized Alzheimer's clinic.

With the tools currently available, physicians can be 85–90% certain about an accurate diagnosis for Alzheimer's.

Some of the more commonly used tests are described below.

Mental State Exams
Mini Mental State Exam (MMSE) — The most widely used and most comprehensive test of cognitive function employed to assist in the diagnosis of Alzheimer's disease. The test may be repeated during the progression of the disease as a measure of decline in cognitive function. The test takes only about 10 minutes to administer and is composed of 11 questions to assess orientation, memory, attention, naming, comprehension, and praxis (customary practice or conduct). The MMSE may not accurately place someone in a particular stage, such as moderate or severe, so this test should be coupled with the clock drawing test and functional activities questionnaire (see below) along with your own observations. MMSEs are ambulatory tests, which means that they can change based on the level of anxiety the test subject feels, the surrounding noise level, the number of people in the room, etc.

26

Physical Self-Maintenance Scale (PSMS) — Tests the patient's ability to perform basic self-maintenance tasks, such as using the toilet, eating, dressing, grooming, bathing, and getting around. The test is given by the caregiver or the doctor during diagnosis and again several times during the course of the disease to monitor change. The patient's scores will increase as the disease progresses.

MATTIS Dementia Rating Scale — Used for detecting neuropsychological impairment and in screening for mild cognitive impairment in the elderly. This diagnostic test addresses social behavior as well as memory impairment.

Global Deterioration Scale — Provides an overview of the stages of cognitive function. Divided into seven stages covering predementia and dementia.

Clock Drawing Task (CDT) — Helpful to differentiate normal elderly persons from those with cognitive impairment and gives an indication that further testing may be warranted. The test is administered by a physician or nurse who asks the subject to draw a clock with the hands pointing to a particular time. The person with memory loss draws a clock that may have the numbers or hands in the wrong places.

In the following illustration, it is easy to see how the CDT helps to identify individuals with a form of dementia. The illustration compares the results from three individuals who were asked to draw a clock showing the time of 10:10 (ten minutes after ten o'clock).

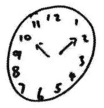 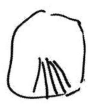

Normal elderly   Mild/moderate   Moderate/severe

The first drawing is from a normal elderly person, the middle drawing is from a person diagnosed with mild to moderate dementia, and the drawing on the right is from a person diagnosed with moderate to severe dementia.

Functional Activities Questionnaire (FAQ) — Particularly useful for an initial assessment of functional impairment. This test is preferred over the MMSE as it allows a more accurate depiction of the subject's loss of ADLs, such as preparing meals, bathing, brushing teeth, etc.

Montreal Cognitive Assessment Test — This is a cognitive screening test designed to help doctors in the diagnosis of Mild Cognitive Impairment. The test is short, about 10 minutes, and assesses attention and concentration, executive functions, memory, language, visuoconstructional skills, conceptual thinking, calculations and orientation.

Diagnostic Imaging

Diagnostic imaging techniques use a variety of devices to take pictures (images) of the human body. Each device has its own strengths and weaknesses in being able to visualize the body's tissues and structures and to help with the process of diagnosis. While these techniques are expensive to use, they provide valuable information to physicians to enable them to make the correct diagnosis. Physicians have several diagnostic imaging devices available to them that are useful in making the diagnosis for Alzheimer's disease. These diagnostic tools include MRI, CT, PET, and SPECT. These are often used with other tests to determine the clinical diagnosis. The PET scan provides the doctor with information about the brain's metabolism. Having this information can improve the doctor's ability to predict the subject's future cognitive functioning by up to 30%. The use of PET may help with earlier diagnosis.

In 2004, Medicare allowed for the reimbursement of the cost of PET scans. However, while PET scans are approved to diagnose frontotemporal dementia, they are not yet approved to diagnose Alzheimer's disease.

Understanding the Diagnosis
You may receive the diagnosis described in one of the following ways:

"Probable Alzheimer's disease or dementia of the Alzheimer's type" — If all the test results appear to be consistent with Alzheimer's.

"Possible Alzheimer's disease" — If the test results indicate that symptoms are not typical for Alzheimer's, but no other diagnosis is found.

If you are unclear about the diagnosis, make sure you ask your doctor, so that you understand and can prepare yourself accordingly.

After the Diagnosis
Once the diagnosis has been made, the physician may or may not develop a health care plan for the person with Alzheimer's disease that will strive to:

o   Maximize functioning and independence.
o   Foster a safe and secure environment.
o   Start medication.
o   Find a support group and other groups that can help the caregiver.
o   Find and enroll in a social model day care facility.

Patient surveillance and health maintenance visits will be scheduled every 3–6 months to:

o   Monitor cognition and behavior with testing.
o   Address and treat comorbid conditions.
o   Evaluate ongoing medications.
o   Check for sleep disturbances.
o   Establish programs to improve behavior and mood.
o   Work closely with family and caregivers.
o   Warn about the hazards of wandering and driving.
o   Encourage modulation of the patient's environment.

If your doctor does not provide you with a health care plan, ask them to do so. If you are unable to discuss this with the doctor at the time of diagnosis, you can make a new appointment to discuss the health care plan specifically.

Now that the diagnosis has been made and you have the plan of care, it is time to start planning and making the decisions that will influence the next few years of your life. You have to plan for your life as a caregiver and you have to plan to take care of yourself while you are fulfilling the caregiver role.

After the diagnosis of Alzheimer's has been made, you are now fully involved in the disease. The individual with Alzheimer's is declining and at times may be more unwilling to listen, comply with directions or health regimes, and may have become sick or need an annual checkup, so you will need to visit the doctor's office regularly. It is important that the person receive regular medical care and you now need to realize that you must plan in advance for a trip to the doctor's office. When making the appointment, find a time with the scheduler that is a time of day that is least crowded, let the office know the person has Alzheimer's, and ask if they can do anything to make the visit easier. Have a friend or family member accompany you to entertain the person while you talk with the doctor or while you wait. Make sure to make the trip enjoyable and plan ample time to leave the house and do not rush. It may be best to tell the person about the appointment shortly before you arrive; be positive, but matter of fact.

Proof of Diagnosis
It is worth noting that the diagnosis of Alzheimer's disease is not foolproof. The only way to prove that Alzheimer's is present is through an autopsy. We encourage caregivers and family members to consider having the autopsy done so that the diagnosis can be confirmed or refuted. This information is valuable in building the family history, particularly for those individuals that have a genetic predisposition to Alzheimer's.

The Many Kinds of Dementia

There are many causes of dementias including those below.

Alzheimer's Disease (AD) — Discovered in 1906 and named after the doctor who made the discovery, Dr. Alois Alzheimer. Alzheimer's disease is a progressive, degenerative brain disease characterized by memory impairment and accompanied by a gradual decline in the patient's ability to perform ADLs, adverse changes in behavior and personality, and a decline in cognitive functions such as language and executive functioning.

Frontotemporal Dementia (FTD) — The term "frontotemporal dementia" refers to a group of diseases that are commonly misdiagnosed as Alzheimer's. We use FTD as a general term to refer to disorders that are also referred to as:

- o Pick's disease
- o Frontotemporal lobar degeneration
- o Progressive aphasia
- o Alcohol-and toxin-induced dementia
- o Diffuse Lewy body dementia
- o Semantic dementia

It is important to identify these individuals early in their course and to refer them to physicians in neurology and psychiatry who are experienced with their management. This referral is primarily important because the clinical course of FTD patients is different than that of patients with Alzheimer's. Patients with FTD have markedly different behavioral manifestations early in the course of disease and appear to have a longer clinical course overall. In addition, when behavioral symptoms predominate, FTD patients who become ill in mid-life may initially be confused with patients with atypical, late-life depression or when the onset is in younger persons, it may be confused with schizophrenia or bipolar disorder.

Creutzfeldt-Jakob Disease (CJD) — A rare and fatal neurodegenerative disease caused by a prion (see Glossary). Patients are usually aged between 50 and 75 and typical clinical features include a rapidly progressive, dementia-associated myoclonus (see Glossary) and a characteristic EEG pattern. Neuropathological examination reveals cortical spongiform change, hence the term "spongiform encephalopathy."

Vascular Dementia/Multi-Infarct Dementia (MID)/Subcortical Ischaemic Vascular Dementia (SIVD) — The second most common form of dementia, ranking after Alzheimer's. The symptoms of vascular dementia are often distinct from those of Alzheimer's. The memory deficits that define Alzheimer's are not always observed in the initial stages of vascular dementia, which is usually characterized by greater impairment of executive function. MID occurs when blood clots block small blood vessels in the brain and destroy brain tissue. As more small vessels are blocked, there is a gradual mental decline. MID, which typically begins between the ages of 60 and 75, affects men more often than women.

Binswanger's Disease — First described by Otto Binswanger in 1894. Binswanger's disease, sometimes referred to as subcortical dementia, is a rare form of dementia characterized by cerebrovascular lesions in the deep white matter of the brain, loss of memory and cognition, and mood changes. It is a slowly progressive condition for which there is no cure. The disorder is often marked by strokes and partial recovery.

Progressive Supranuclear Palsy (PSP) — In people with PSP, gradual loss of certain brain cells causes slowing of movement and reduced control of walking, balance, swallowing, speaking, and eye movement. People with PSP eventually become wheelchair bound or bedridden. PSP is often misdiagnosed as Parkinson's disease because of the general slowing of movement. Less often, it is mistaken for Alzheimer's because of its changes in mood, intellect, and personality.

Alcohol-Induced Dementia/Wernicke-Korsakoff Syndrome — Associated with chronic alcoholism. It also occurs as a complication of gastrointestinal tract disease and complications with malnutrition. This is a degenerative condition of the brain and is caused by a thiamine deficiency. It involves impairment of memory out of proportion to problems with other cognitive functions.

Normal Pressure Hydrocephalus (NPH) — A rare disease caused by an obstruction in the flow of spinal fluid that increases pressure within the cranial cavity and around the brain.

Lewy Body Dementia — Symptoms are similar to a combination of Parkinson's (abnormal movements) and Alzheimer's (dementia) and usually includes hallucinations.

Huntington's Disease — A hereditary disorder characterized by irregular muscle movements, a decline in the ability to think clearly, and other personality changes. This is the only absolute genetic dementia, which is called autosomal, meaning that a child has a 50/50 chance of having the gene that carries the code for Huntington's disease passed on to them by an affected parent.

Traumatic Brain Injury — Brain injuries typically result from accidents in which the head strikes an object. This is the most common type of traumatic brain injury. However, other brain injuries, such as those caused by insufficient oxygen (anoxia), poisoning, or infection can cause similar deficits. Physical deficits can include problems with ambulation, balance, coordination, fine motor skills, strength, and endurance. Cognitive deficits of language and communication, information processing, memory, and perceptual skills are common. Psychological status is also often altered.

Cognitive Impairment After Coronary Bypass Surgery — Cognitive impairment may occur after coronary bypass surgery and is not temporary.

Cognitive Dysfunction in Late-Life Depression (LLD) — Under treated, under recognized, and associated with increased mortality. Patients with LLD show significantly worse performance on tests for memory, speed of responses, language, executive functions, and visuospatial functions as compared with age-and sex-matched controls. Studies support the view that LLD is associated with cognitive impairment. Diseases causing frontostriatal dysfunction in the brain predispose to depression and impairment of executive function; the depression-executive function (DEF) syndrome hypothesis.

Hypoxic-Anoxic Brain Injury — The brain requires a constant flow of oxygen to function normally. A hypoxic-anoxic injury, also known as HAI, occurs when that flow is disrupted, essentially starving the brain and preventing it from performing vital biochemical processes. *Hypoxic* refers to a partial lack of oxygen; *anoxic* means a total lack. In general, the more complete the deprivation, the more severe the harm to the brain and the greater the consequences. The diminished oxygen supply can cause serious impairments in cognitive skills, as well as in physical, psychological, and other functions. Recovery *can* occur in many cases, but it depends largely on the parts of the brain affected and the pace and extent of recovery is unpredictable.

HIV Associated Dementia — also called AIDS dementia complex (ADC), HIV encephalopathy, HIV-1-associated cognitive / motor complex. It is thought to be due to the direct effects of HIV upon the central nervous system (CNS): the brain and spinal cord. Dementia occurs most commonly among people with advanced disease and often progresses rapidly in the absence of HIV treatment.

B12 Deficiency — A deficiency of vitamin B12 often manifests itself first in the development of neurological dysfunction that is almost indistinguishable from senile dementia and Alzheimer's disease. Their symptoms are totally reversible through effective supplementation with vitamin B12.

Neurosyphilis — Dementia, mania or paranoia occurs in about 35% of patients diagnosed with neurosyphilis. The final stage of syphilis, (tertiary stage) occurs in about 15 to 20% of people who have untreated syphilis. Neurosyphilis is a slow progressive, destructive infection of the brain and the spinal cord. The dementia seen in neurosyphilis patients is a progressive dementia characterized by memory problems and disorientation.

4. Symptoms — What to Expect?

By the time the symptoms of Alzheimer's disease are exhibited, the person will have gone through a progressive deterioration, exhibiting some memory loss, declining work performance, concentration deficit, some decline in social skills, denial that anything is wrong with them, and demonstrating anxiety. They may have been diagnosed already with age-associated memory impairment or MCI. As the decline in cognitive function continues, the patient may then be diagnosed as having Alzheimer's and, as we saw in the previous chapter; the diagnosis may be classified as mild, moderate, or severe. In addition to the clinical symptoms the person with Alzheimer's is likely to exhibit, significant changes in behavior are a normal development. While behavioral changes may be very disturbing to the caregiver, family, and friends, they are a direct result of the disease that is slowly incapacitating the patient's brain.

It is impossible to say how long each stage of Alzheimer's will last for each person, but the general pattern is represented below. The symptoms associated with each stage may overlap or may continue from one stage to the next.

Mild Alzheimer's (2–4 years) — In the mild stage of Alzheimer's, the symptoms do not interfere dramatically with everyday life.

o   Forgetfulness, inability to learn new information, memory impairment, decreased knowledge of recent events.
o   Lessening of initiative.
o   Lack of spontaneity.
o   Difficulty managing routine tasks such as finances, planning meals, taking medication on schedule.
o   Depression and terror symptoms.
o   Still able to do most activities, drive car.

Moderate Alzheimer's (2–10 years) — In the moderate stage of Alzheimer's, the patient's ability to think, reason, and function will deteriorate significantly and it is likely that home care or adult day care services will be needed as the person starts to lose the ability to perform daily tasks. The patient can no longer survive without some assistance.

- o Forgetfulness extends to old facts (for example, past career, names of friends).
- o Gets lost going to familiar places, disorientation.
- o Increasing disorientation.
- o Inability to think abstractly.
- o Difficulty performing tasks.
- o Convulsive seizures may develop.
- o Agitation, behavioral symptoms common
  - Restlessness (especially at night), repetitive movements, muscle twitching
  - Wandering
  - Paranoia, delusions, hallucinations.
- o Deficits in intellect and reasoning (for example, poor judgment, forgets manners).
- o Decreasing concern for appearance, hygiene, and sleep becomes more noticeable.

Severe Alzheimer's (1–3 years) — In the final stage of Alzheimer's, the patient requires full-time care.

- o Unable to use or understand words.
- o Total disorientation.
- o May groan, scream, mumble, or speak gibberish.
- o Behavioral symptoms common
  - Refuses to eat
  - Inappropriately cries out.
- o Failure to recognize family or faces (including their own).
- o Difficulty with essential ADLs (for example, unable to bathe, incontinent).

People with advanced Alzheimer's are most likely to:

- o Need help walking and eventually become bedridden or chair bound.
- o Find it difficult to eat or swallow.

o   Be at risk for infections and pneumonia.
o   Lose the ability to communicate with words.
o   Need full-time care with everything, including toileting.

Changes in Behavior

The changes in behavior that will be exhibited in the individual with Alzheimer's disease can be the most difficult for the caregiver to manage. You are still involved with your own social environment, you have your own friends, and yet you have accepted the responsibility to be a caregiver. Now you are going to be put in difficult situations and possibly embarrassed and humiliated in front of your family and friends (as well as in front of strangers) because of the individual's use of inappropriate language, sexual acts, or other socially unacceptable behavior. It is time for you to try to understand what is happening to them as their memory declines and they forget how to behave. After all, you do not want to shut them away from the outside world, so it becomes necessary to find ways to deal with the behavioral problems you will encounter. It is essential to remember that you should not try to correct their behavior, as this will create anxiety or agitation. In any case, they are more likely to believe that you are the one that is wrong if you do try to correct them. Rather, you should redirect them to do something more appropriate that has purpose and can occupy them. The person with Alzheimer's cannot logically understand that their behavior may be inappropriate.

They may exhibit strong emotions, resulting in challenging behavior that may become more frequent and severe. When these situations arise, it is important to listen to them and understand the cause of the emotions so that you can try to redirect them to a more acceptable behavior, especially when you are in public. If they exhibit signs of depression, your physician should be consulted as soon as possible so that the depression can be treated. Depression occurs in about 40% of Alzheimer's patients and is a serious matter as it can exacerbate the symptoms of dementia and cause a more profound pseudodementia that may result in the person appearing more impaired than they actually are. By treating the depression, you will improve their quality of life.

General Problems of Behavior

- o Denial of problems.
- o Wandering, sleep disturbances.
- o Sundowner's Syndrome (behavior worsens in the evening) marked by obsessive or repetitious behaviors, anger, agitation, or crying.
- o Inappropriate sexual behavior/comments.
- o Losing/hiding things.
- o Repetitious actions/questions.
- o Clinging behavior (following you around everywhere).
- o Complaints, insults, demanding things.
- o Throwing and breaking items.
- o Giving money or personal items away to strangers, family, or friends.
- o Isolation or stating that they do not want to go out.
- o Lack of personal hygiene.
- o Disrobing or going outside naked.
- o Pinching, spitting, biting.

General Problems of Mood

- o Depression, suicidal thoughts or feelings.
- o Apathy or listlessness.
- o Anger, agitation, anxiety, restlessness.
- o False ideas and beliefs (delusions).
- o Suspiciousness and accusing others.
- o Crying, sobbing, crying out.
- o Paranoia.
- o Hallucinations (a person may see, hear, feel, or smell things that are not there).
- o Delusions (addressing figments of the imagination as if they were real).
- o Misinterpretation (of actions, events, conversations).

While these behavioral changes can be difficult for you to manage, they are a result of the neuronal degeneration caused by the disease. We have selected a few of the more common behavioral changes to comment on that you should be aware of and that require particular patience and understanding on your part, as you may be embarrassed, humiliated, and otherwise publicly shamed by the person with Alzheimer's disease. It is always important for you to remember that they cannot control the way they behave. The part of their brain that once controlled impulse and consequence/action no longer exists. Trying to argue with the person with Alzheimer's will get you nowhere. This disease rips away the ability for the individual to reason and have cognitive thought. Therefore, to better manage the behavioral problems you will face, you should concede that the person with Alzheimer's is right 100% of the time, even when you know they are wrong. In this way, you will be able to redirect their behavior to something more appropriate. They are living in quite a different world than you or I.

Through the mild and moderate stages of Alzheimer's, the patient certainly has some awareness that they are in cognitive decline, even if they are in denial that the problems really exist. They will also have some awareness that they have to be cared for and they may believe they are becoming a burden on the caregiver and their family. In this situation, they can delude themselves into thinking that they are going to be abandoned or institutionalized and that the caregiver no longer wants to take care of them. Unfortunately, they cannot remember how much you are really doing for them.

Because the person with Alzheimer's cannot be convinced that they will not be abandoned, they may also believe that the caregiver has become unfaithful to them either in the more intimate sexual sense or in the more general caregiver sense. They may develop such a fear or phobia of being left alone that their anxiety levels rise when the caregiver leaves the room or goes out of their sight. Abandonment is the most basic of emotions and relates back to childhood. The best thing you can do is to reassure them of how they are needed in your life to help you and celebrate the love and happiness they give you. Always remember, a smile and a hug, even when they have lashed out. It is the disease talking, not them.

Falling and Problems with Balance
About one-third of people with moderate to severe Alzheimer's disease fall on a regular basis and the rate of falling is a symptom of the severity of their disease.

Balance can be an issue for the person with Alzheimer's disease, leading to an unsteady gait and an increased risk for falls to occur. The balance issue can be caused by various factors, such as changes in the body/brain, medications (such as Resperidol / Residperidone / Haldol), inner ear infections, and a quick fall in blood pressure (if the person stands up too quickly). If you suspect a balance issue, consult your physician. Within three years of diagnosis about half of all patients report problems with gait.

Weight Loss
Weight loss is a symptom of Alzheimer's disease and a loss of weight may be an early indicator of the disease. The simple act of weighing yourself or insisting that you be weighed when you visit your doctor so that a history of your weight gains and losses are recorded may cause your doctor to look at Alzheimer's disease as a possible cause especially if there is no other obvious reason for the weight loss.

It has been known for a long time that people with Alzheimer's disease tend to be thinner than their healthy counterparts and weight loss can become substantial as the disease progresses. Research studies have shown that men who develop dementia in later life will start to lose weight about six years before their diagnosis of Alzheimer's disease when compared to men who do not develop the disease. Their rate of weight loss increases in the three years before diagnosis. So it is reasonable to suspect that changes occurring in the brain as MCI and then Alzheimer's develops are having an effect on appetite and other causes resulting in weight loss.

Sundowner's Syndrome
One of the characteristics of Alzheimer's disease is that the individual may have more behavioral problems in the evening. This may be because they have been awake and "active" all day and they become overwhelmed by the time evening comes. By "sundown" they are not able to cope as well with the confusing environment around them. They may become increasingly confused, agitated, and anxious and may pace the floor, begin to wander, or show other nervous behaviors.

To help minimize Sundowner's Syndrome, maintain a structured daily routine. This reduces the anxiety that decision making can produce. Scheduled rest periods should be included in that routine. Try to keep the daily activities within the person's coping ability. Surprises, challenges, or a lot of new information can be very upsetting. Special occasions, outings, family visits, and other changes in routine should be explained in advance and approached gently. It is best to schedule these events after quiet days. Turn lights on inside the house well before dusk to lessen disorientation.

Catastrophic Reactions

Catastrophic reactions occur when the person with Alzheimer's disease is out of their routine or a situation overwhelms their thinking capacity. The behaviors that result may include anger, crying, wandering, pacing, agitation, lashing out, rapidly changing mood, paranoia, blushing, or stubbornness. When these behaviors occur, try to validate their feelings and then redirect them to an activity they enjoy.

5. Time for Planning

Now that Alzheimer's disease has been diagnosed, it is time to make some decisions and start planning for the future. The role of the caregiver will be totally consuming and it is essential that the caregiver plan to take care of themselves as well as the patient. Do not forget yourself — you, the caregiver! Burnout can creep up out of the blue if you do not take care of yourself and plan for your own well being.

The first crucial decision is to decide who will be the primary caregiver. Frequently, this will be the spouse, but if no spouse is available or if the spouse is unable to cope with the responsibilities of being a caregiver to an Alzheimer's patient, then an alternative caregiver will be needed, either a family member or, perhaps, a friend. You may decide to consult your physician to obtain a medical opinion as to your suitability to serve as a caregiver.

Frequently, of course, there is no choice. You are the spouse and nobody else is stepping forward. You do not feel that you can abandon your partner of many years and so, like it or not, you are it. Make the most of it. Learn to enjoy the few years left together and plan carefully to make sure that you can do the very best for you both.

Whoever the caregiver is, they will need to build their own support group from family members, friends, and external groups. More of this later.

From what you have read already, you know that the average life expectancy for the Alzheimer's patient is around 8 years after diagnosis. Some patients will survive less time and some will survive as much as 20 years or more. Statistics gathered on Alzheimer's patients show that 75% will be moved to a nursing home or other facility after 5 years. So without making the planning process too complex, we have prepared some guidelines to help you.

What is the point of planning? Planning helps to take out the uncertainty about the future. Planning makes you do your homework so that you will be able to identify potential problem areas and solve them in a timely manner. Planning will help you to gather the information you need so that you make the best decisions for the person with Alzheimer's and for yourself.

As the disease progresses, the patient will require constant supervision, making caregiving a full-time job. Since 35% of all caregivers work outside the home, it becomes necessary either to arrange for professional care or for the caregiver to stop working and stay with the patient. In either case, the costs are considerable and planning for this eventuality is essential.

There are many practical issues for which you will have to plan including financial, legal, safety, etc. One of the most important for you, the caregiver, is time. Planning your time can make the difference between coping and not coping. Setting routine for the patient, while ensuring that you have time for yourself, is essential for you to lead a decent life.

For most people, financial planning will be a key concern and an area on which to focus. You should expect that the cost of caring for the Alzheimer's patient will be on the order of $120,000 or perhaps much more over the remaining life of the patient. The most expensive part will be the cost of care in a nursing home or other facility in the last few years of the patient's life. Recent reports suggest that the cost of a year in a nursing home is $57,500 and part-time care can cost as much as $26,000. However, there are other matters that require planning and the caregiver's attention, such as legal matters, therapy, moving, and contingency planning. What happens if something happens to you, the caregiver? Who will take your place?

We know that the individual's symptoms will get worse with time and they will become more dependent on the caregiver to the point that they will be totally dependent. As soon as the diagnosis is known, start the planning process to optimize available treatments and services and to ease the burden on you.

Once again, we emphasize the importance of an early diagnosis. While the patient is still aware and can make their wishes known, involve them as much as possible in the planning process. If you are not the one who paid the bills, arranged the finances, or took care of legal matters, you will have to learn these things and it will be much easier if the patient is able to participate.

As part of the planning process, you should start by educating yourself about Alzheimer's. Learn what happens as the disease progresses and learn how to deal with the patient in an effective manner. Remember, the patient is not going to be in control of what they do; the disease will take over their cognitive functioning. You, the caregiver, are the one who must change to meet the patient's needs. Your communication style, attitudes, and ability to fill the patient's needs will be reflected in the well being and behaviors of the patient. There are many websites that can provide information on Alzheimer's and we list some of these later in this book. Also, there are local and national associations that provide useful information and support for caregivers. This book will give you some of the guidance you need.

Financial and legal issues will play an important part in caring for the Alzheimer's patient and these issues should be tended to immediately. Discuss as much as possible with your loved one while they are still able to help you. If your family has an accountant, lawyer, financial planner, or other professional that has assisted you previously, identify them and locate their respective files and records. You should then contact each of these professionals to apprise them of the patient's condition and seek their advice. If you think it necessary, perhaps because your home records are incomplete or if you are not sure if they are complete, arrange to meet with the professionals so that you can become fully informed of the relevant financial and legal issues. It is not uncommon for spouses not to know of their financial status. They have been happy to leave financial and legal matters to their partner. This has to change. The caregiver must now be the person that is fully informed and starting to make the decisions on these critical issues.

If financial and legal professionals have not been involved with the patient's affairs, you must decide if you have the ability to take on the responsibility of managing the household finances and any legal issues. If you do not feel sufficiently knowledgeable to take this on, talk to family members, maybe they can help. If you want professional help, ask for recommendations from friends who have had positive experiences with particular accountants, lawyers, and others.

You know that the person with Alzheimer's will go through stages of decline over a period of years. Eventually, they will die from Alzheimer's or another disease. There are certain items that are very important to have in place so that there is no ambiguity about what to do in the late stages and after the death of the patient. Preferably, these legal documents should be drawn up while the patient is still competent to have a say in the way their affairs will be handled, particularly the way they want to be treated when they are no longer in control of their cognitive functions. If you do not have these legal documents already in place, we recommend that you visit an attorney, either your family attorney or an attorney experienced in elder affairs, at the earliest opportunity.

The key documents to consider having in place while the patient is still competent are a will, medical and durable power of attorney, living will, health care surrogate, conservator, and do not resuscitate (DNR) order. Discuss these documents with your attorney to determine which are most appropriate for you and for the state in which you live.

These documents will establish your ability to make financial, legal, and medical decisions for the person with Alzheimer's when they can no longer make rational or calculated decisions themselves. There are distinct differences between each of these documents, all of which should be prepared with the assistance of an attorney.

- o A durable power of attorney (or POA) is a legal document that authorizes you, the caregiver, to either have financial power of attorney, health care power of attorney, or both, depending on how it is written. If you have both, a POA will allow you the ability to make all legal, health (treatment), caregiving, and financial decisions on behalf of the person with Alzheimer's.

o The surrogate becomes the attorney-in-fact, and any competent adult can be selected to be the surrogate, although a member of the medical team should not be selected because of possible conflicts of interest. Select just one person to be the surrogate, although others may be selected to serve as alternates in the event the chosen person is unavailable or unable to make decisions. Surrogates cannot be held liable for decisions made regarding the patient's care or for costs associated with medical care. The surrogate can only make decisions when the patient is temporarily or permanently unable to make their own health care decisions.

o A conservator handles all the legal oversight and decisions for health care in the person's best interest and is appointed by the court. A conservator can be a professional conservator (third party) or it can be a friend or family member who seeks consevatorship from the court.

o A living will establishes the wants and desires of the individual who authors the document. This may establish the health issues of the person and may include a DNR order.

o A DNR establishes the wishes that a person not have CPR performed in case of a heart attack or other accident or condition that may require CPR.

o A will establishes all of the wishes of an individual, which may include designating a POA in case of incapacitation, will include dispersement of assets, and could possibly contain the living will.

The next key issue is financial. It is vital that you identify and plan how to manage financial resources to recognize how monies should be spent and where there might be insufficient funds. The caregiver may be responsible for paying bills, arranging for benefit claims, investment decisions, tax returns, etc.

The first step is to locate and identify financial and insurance documents, such as insurance policies (life, long-term care, disability, health, auto, homeowners), investments, bank accounts, pension and other retirement benefits, Social Security payments, other forms of income, deeds or mortgage papers, or ownership statements and bills. If you are uncertain what to do and your loved one cannot help, involve a family member who is more familiar with taking care of the financial responsibilities in their own household. You will quickly learn to take care of the details and make the decisions yourself. It is essential that you make sure that you have access to all the funds of the patient. If you are the spouse and you did not have joint bank accounts, joint investments, etc., you must make sure that the accounts are changed so that you have access to the funds. Do this while the patient is competent so that you do not have to go through more complicated and possibly costly procedures later.

Once you have determined that you have access to all the funds and insurance policies, you can start to make some calculations for what your income and expenses are going to be. Do not forget the equity that you may have in your home that can be turned into cash through loans, lines of credit, or a reverse mortgage.

Keep in mind that if you, the caregiver, are currently working and earning, you will either eventually have to give up your job to take care of the patient or pay for someone else to do it, unless there is another family member or friend who can care for the patient without pay while you are at work. Do not underestimate the burden on yourself as you will have to decide if you are able to both work and take care of the patient when you come home.

Once you have an overview of the financial situation, you will be able to make a determination if there are sufficient financial resources to cover the cost of care. If you find there are sufficient funds available, you want to make sure that your financial resources are protected. This is probably not the time for you to be investing in high-risk ventures, but look for a more conservative approach that will protect your capital and give you an acceptable level of return on your investments. A financial advisor can help you if you are not comfortable making these kinds of decisions.

If you find that you will not have the financial resources to take care of the patient or if you believe it will be very tight, you should start to look for other sources of financial support. Do you have any funds not already included in your calculations? Approach family members with your appraisal of the financial situation and get their input as to ways to help out. How much can they contribute? Are there friends that were close enough to you or your loved one that might want to help?

To help you to obtain a realistic estimate of the cost of long-term care, it is a good idea to call several adult day care facilities, respite services, specialized assisted living communities, and local nursing homes with Alzheimer's facilities to find out their costs and what their projections are for cost increases. This knowledge will help you to project the cost of the last few years of the patient's life more accurately. Even though you may now say that you will never put your loved one in a nursing home or other facility, the burden on the caregiver is a heavy one and you may no longer be able to cope after several years of caring. Remember, 75% of patients go into nursing homes and other facilities 5 years after diagnosis, so it is better that you plan financially to have the money available for a facility even if you ultimately do not use it.

Now what about you? What will happen to the patient if something happens to you and you are no longer able to take care of them? Make contingency plans and look into taking out (more) insurance on yourself to provide a financial safety net for yourself and those dependent on your income. Disability and life insurance should be considered, but talk to an insurance agent or a financial planner to see what may be best in your particular situation.

Find out if there is a family member or friend who will take over the role of caregiver if something should happen to you. If there is, make sure that you put the necessary legal documents in place to give them access to your assets and that they are named as caregiver/guardian. Consult an attorney about this. Remember, you could be in an accident tomorrow and you must make sure that you and your loved one are taken care of.

Budgeting

Knowing how much money is coming in (income) whether from jobs, investments, or other sources and knowing how much money is being spent (expenses) in the patient's household is essential for most people. Keep good records and prepare a budget for yourself. There are several good computer programs around that do this in a very structured way, but if you prefer pen and paper, keep track of the items of expense and income so you always know what your financial situation is and, just as important, you make it possible for someone else to find out the financial situation if anything happens to you.

When budgeting, take into account what insurance benefits the patient may have. Are they eligible for Medicare or Medicaid? If so, is there Medigap insurance in place and, if not, does it make financial sense to get Medigap insurance? Does the patient have disability insurance that comes into effect? Is there long-term care insurance? Is there life insurance that could be used to provide cash? Are there any other retirement plans? What Social Security benefits does the patient receive? Is the patient eligible for Social Security disability income, supplemental security income, veteran's benefits, or any tax benefits? You may be eligible for medical expense deductions and dependent care credits on your tax return.

If the patient is still able to work, what employee benefits are there?

More Planning

Now that you have taken care of financial and legal matters, you should turn your attention to planning your daily life and that of the patient. Your life as the caregiver will change; there is no doubt about that. If you plan your days and live a more structured life than you may otherwise have done, you will also be able to plan for yourself, for the time you will need for yourself.

The person with Alzheimer's disease needs help. As the disease gets worse, the patient needs more help. This is the way it is. You must establish routines for them and for yourself to minimize stress on you both.

Recognizing what help they need will help you to plan your days. As their condition changes, you may have to change your daily plans to accommodate those changes. Remember, it is you who must change; they are not capable of changing to accommodate your needs. They are dependent on you to guide and cue them.

As a start, identify their needs and make the time available to take care of each one. In the mild stages, they may need help dressing, seeing to personal care, doing chores, making meals, meeting friends, or going out. It is important to plan activities into their daily lives so that they can retain a sense of purpose and dignity. Set up a routine for them and give them something to look forward to. Activities may be with friends, with you, or, if possible, alone. Activities should be planned to help them use the abilities they have left. This will vary from patient to patient, but plan activities where the patient is involved and achieving something, and where they can receive positive feedback. Include physical exercises such as walking; intellectual activities such as reading, crossword puzzles, and jigsaw puzzles; creative activities such as music, painting, and writing; and any hobbies they are able to pursue. If the patient is a religious or spiritual person, involve their religious organization.

Your role in their activities is to give support, encouragement, help when needed, and supervision. You should be aware of their limitations and encourage them to do things at which they are able to succeed and enjoy. Keep things simple and be patient with them so that they are able to enjoy what they are doing. Remember, this is about them and not about you. While planning the activities, consider things that help them to remain independent and plan the activities so that distractions are minimized and you can control the environment so that they do not become frightened or confused. Plan activities in familiar surroundings. Once you learn what the patient enjoys, you can modify the planned activities to maximize their enjoyment and participation.

Do not avoid spontaneous activities such as trips or going out to dinner as long as the patient's behavior is appropriate. Involvement in activities may also help to keep them occupied rather than indulging in less-desirable behaviors such as wandering off or being agitated or anxious. Planning activities for the patient is also beneficial for the caregiver. You know where the patient is, so you do not have to worry about them. You can see them having fun participating with friends, other patients, or you. Being assured as to their safety and well being helps to reduce your own stress.

Safety
As the disease progresses and the cognitive function of the patient declines, their immediate surroundings can become a dangerous place if precautions are not taken. It is time to look at the patient's residence and make safe anything that could be considered dangerous or might even be used as a weapon. More guidance on safety matters is provided in Chapter 7.

Moving
One of the key decisions the caregiver and the patient's family will have to make is to determine at what point it is no longer possible for the caregiver to look after the patient. Circumstances vary widely depending on the condition of the patient, the ability of the caregiver, finances, etc. It is useful to make a determination in advance when you think a move might be necessary, so that you can research suitable care facilities and communicate with family members and the health care team.

Planning for the End
While this can be a difficult topic to discuss, there should be no doubt in the minds of the caregiver and family members that the patient will die, directly or indirectly, as a result of Alzheimer's disease. Eventually, you will have to assume full responsibility for the loved one's affairs.

Encourage the patient, as soon as possible after diagnosis, to select an advance directive (either a living will or a durable POA) that expresses their wishes for treatment at the end of their life. It is important to use the advance directive form(s) recognized by the state in which care will be provided. If no advance directive is drawn up, it may be advisable to consult an attorney for advice on how to proceed, as there are other options (such as conservatorship) that may better serve the patient.

Become familiar with the range of medical care available:

- o Treatment strategies.
- o Aggressive care.
- o Feeding tubes and IV hydration.
- o Conservative care.
- o Palliative care.

Be prepared to make decisions.

- o Be guided by the person's wishes and preferences.
- o Work with family members and the health care team.
- o Consider using a trusted third party to facilitate the decision-making process.

Resolving Family Conflicts

Be prepared for family conflicts. There may well be opinions from family members about how to manage the end of the person's life, even when there are legal documents in place that describe the person's wishes. Make sure that you have the legal documents in place that make it clear who has the decision-making responsibility. If the conflict becomes unmanageable for you, consider involving a third party who understands the law and the person's wishes, and can help to defuse a difficult situation.

After Death

When the patient eventually dies, many caregivers feel a great sense of relief. The burden of caregiving is over. Do not feel guilty about having this reaction as it is very common and understandable. Your own normal life can now resume without the need to care for another, and you may find that your health improves, particularly if you have been depressed. There are many reports of caregivers experiencing rapid recovery from depression after the death of the person they have been caring for.

About 90% of caregivers surveyed felt their patient was relieved to have died and many believe their patient was in pain before they died. Thus, it can be considered a relief to everyone that it is finally over.

Planning for You

Your role of caregiver will be demanding and there will be times when you feel that you cannot cope. In Chapter 7, we present some tips and tools for caregivers that we believe will help you in your daily life as a caregiver. It will help you if you structure your life and plan your day so there is time for you to pursue what you enjoy, whether it is reading, meeting friends, watching television, hobbies, or whatever else can help you to relax and enjoy your own life. Find out what resources are available in your community. There are options available to help both you and the patient. Consider attending a support group and learn how to care for yourself as a caregiver. Also, consider using social model day care and overnight respite services in order to give you some time for yourself to recharge your batteries. A stressed, overtired caregiver cannot provide the type of care they are trying so hard to give.

If you decide to continue working after the person has been diagnosed with Alzheimer's disease, you will have to plan for day care with family, friends, or with a day care facility. Your time with the Alzheimer's patient will then be planned around your work schedule. Even though you will have just a few hours to work with, make sure that you establish the routine for the individual and make sure that you plan some time for yourself.

6. Therapies

For the patient and the caregiver, you should learn from your doctor all the therapies available for the treatment of Alzheimer's disease. In some instances, you may have to insist on receiving the information because some doctors do not believe the drug therapies work and may not want to burden you with the cost of these therapies. However, we believe that you should be informed so that you can participate in the decision making about what therapies should be pursued. Some treatment is better than no treatment at all. Once you start to give the drug prescribed by your doctor, it is essential that you continue to administer the drugs even if you are not seeing real improvements, because the drugs may be slowing the progression of the disease.

So why is it that some members of the medical profession believe that the drugs do not work? We believe that part of the problem arises from the fact that none of the available drugs cure the disease nor do they necessarily improve the symptoms of the patient. We believe the other part is due to the need for education of some doctors as to the benefits of drug therapies in Alzheimer's.

To explore this topic further, we need to go back to the description of Alzheimer's as a progressive, incurable disease. The fact that Alzheimer's is described as progressive implies that the course of the disease is on a time line and that the cognitive functions and memory loss in the patient continue to decline as the patient moves along the time line, that is, as they get older. If we accept that there is no cure and that symptoms are not necessarily improved by available drugs, what other benefits might the drugs have? The answer is that the drugs may be effective in delaying the progression of the disease. They rarely stop the progression of the disease, but they can delay the progression to such an extent that the life of the patient and the caregiver are impacted positively. Several studies have been conducted by researchers and clinicians that confirm the positive actions of these drugs.

If the available drugs are able to impact the lives of the patient and the caregiver positively, it makes sense that there is also a positive economic effect for the patient's family as well as for society in general. This so-called pharmacoeconomic benefit needs further explanation, as one of the arguments for not prescribing drugs to Alzheimer's patients is the cost of the drugs themselves. Various studies have been conducted that have produced similar findings that the use of drugs delays the progression of the disease and reduces the immediate cost of care. If we take into account that, on average, the first symptoms of Alzheimer's appear at 75 years of age and we are able to delay, through drug or other therapy, the appearance of the first symptoms of Alzheimer's, this would mean that roughly 50% of the individuals would die of other causes without ever suffering the effects of Alzheimer's.

In making these calculations, the cost to the caregiver is important when you consider the number of workdays lost and the number of hours spent caring for the patient (caregivers spend an average of 85 hours a week caring for their patient).

If you can imagine that your loved one has been diagnosed with Alzheimer's and they still retain sufficient use of their memory and cognitive functions to recognize you and be useful around the house, go out with you, etc., would you not rather prolong them in that state as long as possible rather than see them deteriorate at a much faster rate? Each ADL that the patient loses has a cost associated with it in terms of the extra care and attention the patient needs. The more the patient is able to do for themselves, the more satisfying for both patient and caregiver and the immediate cost of care is reduced. The lowered cost to the family can be in the order of one to several thousand dollars per year, and if we consider that even 5 million Americans are diagnosed with Alzheimer's and two-thirds to three-quarters are not prescribed drug therapy, the savings to American society every year is already in the billions of dollars.

There is no doubt that as the disease worsens the cost to both patient and caregiver rises dramatically in terms of health care costs and lost productivity of caregivers. A recent study at UCLA showed that health care costs totaled approximately $20,000 in a 6-month period compared to $35,000 for patients with severe dementia during the same period, leading one to conclude that treatment to slow the progression of the disease may help lower costs. Just as important or perhaps more important, it has been shown that the time doctors have to spend with patients treated with medications is significantly less than untreated patients and that the burden on the caregiver is less and nursing home placement may be delayed in treated patients.

What are the Available Therapies?
There are no therapies proven to slow the onset of Alzheimer's disease but available therapies can slow the disease's progression, and maximize the functioning of the remaining active neurons. For high-risk groups that have not been diagnosed with Alzheimer's disease, there are some treatments that can be considered to slow the onset or progression of the disease. Several categories of such therapies are available: (1) estrogen for women, (2) nonsteroidal anti-inflammatory medications, (3) antioxidants (for example, vitamin E that has recently been shown to be involved in the regulating genes that, in turn, regulate hormones and hormone metabolism, nerve growth factors, apoptosis [cell death], and the clearance of beta amyloid in animal studies), and (4) treatments for other conditions such as depression that can result in a higher incidence of Alzheimer's. Each has potential, minor benefits in slowing the onset or progression of symptoms, but none will stop the disease.

Estrogen Therapy
Estrogen therapy for dementias is controversial at best. In some recent studies, estrogen has been shown to increase dementia and heart disease. Current thinking is to use estrogen only for the symptoms of menopause and not for the prevention of dementia and heart disease.

Earlier studies have shown that women who receive estrogen replacements after menopause may have lower rates of Alzheimer's disease and slower rates of intellectual loss when compared to women who receive no hormone replacement. However, the use of estrogen in postmenopausal women may increase the likelihood for breast cancer and surgical removal of the uterus for abnormal bleeding or uterine malignancy. Women with a strong family history for Alzheimer's should discuss the benefits versus the risks of estrogen replacements with a physician who understands the use of this medication and its role in preventing age-related complications in the brain, bone, and heart.

Testosterone Therapy in Men

Some studies suggest that a gel containing the hormone testosterone could have a beneficial effect on the mood, energy level and overall physical health in men with Alzheimer's disease. However the testosterone gel, rubbed into the skin, does not seem to improve memory or other mental processes. You should consult your doctor about the possible benefits of testosterone replacement therapy for male patients.

Anti-Inflammatory Medications

Although inflammation is not a major part of Alzheimer's disease, an inflammatory response is part of the damage that occurs in the Alzheimer's brain.

Patients who receive continuous doses of nonsteroidal anti-inflammatory drugs (NSAIDs), such as aspirin, acetaminophen, and ibuprofen, may have lower rates of dementia and slower rates of cognitive decline than individuals who do not receive this medication, although recent studies of two of these drugs, rofecoxib (Vioxx, which is no longer available) and naproxen (Aleve), have shown that they did not delay the progression of Alzheimer's in people who already have the disease.

Antioxidants

Antioxidants are substances that absorb free radicals in the brain (and other parts of the body) or retard the production of these harmful substances. A wide range of normally occurring substances and pharmacological agents will reduce free radical production in the brain. Individuals who consume high levels of antioxidant substances such as beta-carotene have less intellectual decline with aging. High doses of vitamin E (that is, 1,000–2,000 units per day) may slow the onset of Alzheimer's disease and the progression of intellectual loss. However, there are possible cardiovascular risks at doses above 400 units per day and you should follow your physician's directions. Vitamin E is the most widely discussed free radical scavenger and substantial doses are required for protective effect. The long-term consequences of high doses of vitamin E are not understood and the duration of brain protection is unknown. Other substances also have free radical protection, including vitamin C and the medication selegiline. Patients at high risk for developing dementia (for example, individuals over the age of 65 with family histories of Alzheimer's) may consider long-term use of vitamin E, but it is essential that you discuss this with your doctor so you can better understand the possible risks. Dementia experts neither encourage nor discourage the use of this vitamin. Gingko biloba may also act by absorbing free radicals, although other protective effects may occur with this medication. There is no clear clinical evidence to support the use of Gingko biloba to prevent dementia. A 2007 report from a study in France of 3,534 men and women aged 65 and older concluded that taking Gingko had no effect on the likelihood of developing dementia. The long-term side effect of Gingko in elderly individuals is unknown, although this medicine has been widely used in Europe for many decades without clear, long-term, serious side effects.

For patients who have Alzheimer's disease you might consider giving high dose vitamin E (1,000 units twice a day) based upon a large-scale clinical trial that showed slowing of progression of the disease. You may add high dose vitamin C (1,000 mg per day). Discuss with your physician before taking these supplements.

Antidepressants
Older people with persistent depression are at higher risk for developing dementia. Untreated depression produces cognitive loss and functional decline in older patients. Depressed elders should be aggressively treated for depression to minimize physical and intellectual complications from a disease that usually responds to antidepressant medications.

Drug Therapies
At the present time, the medications most effective in the therapy of Alzheimer's disease work by altering the chemical balance in the neurons of selected areas of the brain. In Alzheimer's, the brain's neurons are damaged such that the chemicals (neurotransmitters) that are responsible for passing messages between neurons are adversely affected (a more complete description of the scientific and

medical basis of Alzheimer's can be found in Chapter 9). The effective medications try to bring the neurotransmitters back into balance. While several neurotransmitters are found in the brain, it is the manipulation of two of these, acetylcholine and glutamate, which has so far shown a positive effect in Alzheimer's patients. The classes of drugs are known as acetylcholinesterase (AChE) inhibitors and NMDA (N-methyl-D-aspartate) receptor antagonists, respectively. The former appear to be more effective in mild to moderate and the latter more effective in moderate to severe Alzheimer's although Aricept, an AChE inhibitor, was approved recently in the US for the treatment of severe Alzheimer's disease as well as mild and moderate Alzheimer's. Acetylcholine concentrations have been shown to fall sharply in people with Alzheimer's. AChE is an enzyme that is responsible for the natural breakdown of acetylcholine and inhibition of the enzyme will raise the levels of acetylcholine available to the neurons. Examples of AChE inhibitors used in the treatment of Alzheimer's are Donepezil HCL (Aricept), Rivastigmine tartrate (Exelon), Galantamine HBr (Reminyl and Razadyne ER), and Tacrine HCl (Cognex), which is no longer prescribed.

Use of these drugs has been shown to either improve or slow the decline of cognitive functions, such as memory, thinking, and everyday activities such as eating and dressing in some patients with Alzheimer's as well as reduce behavioral disturbances.

By treating with cholinesterase inhibitors, one can preserve functioning at home for at least one year. Given the costs of being in residential care, this is a tremendous benefit. In addition to the cost, it is a benefit to the family to have someone functioning well enough to be at home for additional years.

NMDA receptor antagonists are used to treat the symptoms of moderate to severe Alzheimer's. These drugs block the activity of glutamate in the brain. Glutamate is important in memory and learning and is released in abnormal amounts in people with Alzheimer's, causing damage to brain cells. Only one drug in this class, Memantine HCL (Namenda), is currently available to be prescribed. Namenda is the only treatment indicated for people with moderate to severe Alzheimer's and may help with memory, behavior, and the ability to do daily tasks over a period of time.

Don't Stop Taking the Drugs

It is very important that patients take their medication as prescribed, and continue to take the medication unless side effects become intolerable, in which case consult your doctor so that an alternative drug can be prescribed since patients unable to tolerate one drug are often able to tolerate an alternative medication. We cannot emphasize enough the need for therapy to be maintained as prescribed by your doctor so that the full benefits of drug therapy can be realized. If drug therapy is interrupted, the benefits of slowing the progression of the disease may be lost

It is up to the caregiver to ensure medications are taken as prescribed. The patient may forget to take the medication or may take several doses because they forget they have already taken it. Even though you may not see much improvement in the patient's symptoms, the drugs are acting to slow the progression of the disease and continued medication is necessary to retain any benefits the medications may provide.

Prescription Drugs

Prescription drugs should only be taken according to your doctor's instructions. If you are taking other medications, make sure you inform your doctor since this information will help him/her determine any possible drug interactions.

Though not a cure, the drugs approved for the treatment of Alzheimer's disease have been shown to be effective in slowing the progression of and treating the symptoms of the disease. It is important for you to monitor your patient's behavior and response to the medication and stay in touch with your doctor because strategic prescription changes and dosage adjustments can keep the person with Alzheimer's disease stable for years.

Aricept® (Donepezil HCl) is the first drug to receive FDA approval for all stages (mild, moderate and severe) of Alzheimer's disease and is one of the class of drugs called acetylcholinesterase inhibitors (see chapter 9 for more information). As well as providing symptomatic relief in patients with Alzheimer's disease, Aricept has been shown to slow the rate of brain shrinkage in patients with MCI and who carry the APOE4 gene (See chapter 9).

Aricept comes in 2 different strengths (5 mg and 10 mg). Your doctor may suggest 5 mg, once a day, for the first 4 to 6 weeks of treatment and then, once your patient adjusts to the medication, the doctor may increase the dose to 10 mg once a day. Aricept can be taken with or without food.

Some of the side effects of Aricept include nausea, diarrhea, not sleeping well (especially if taken at bedtime), vomiting, muscle cramps, feeling very tired, or not wanting to eat. Other side effects may occur. Inform your doctor of any side effects as he/she may want to adjust the dose or consider an alternative medication. People at risk for ulcers should tell their doctors because their condition may get worse. More information on Aricept can be found on the website www.aricept.com.

Exelon® (Rivastigmine tartrate) is available as pills and in an oral solution and is indicated for mild to moderate Alzheimer's disease. It is also one of the class of drugs called acetylcholinesterase inhibitors (see chapter 9 for more information).

The dosage of Exelon shown to be effective is 6-12 mg/day, given twice a day (BID) (daily doses of 3 to 6 mg BID). There is some evidence that doses at the higher end of this range may be more beneficial.

The starting dose of Exelon is 1.5 mg BID. If this dose is well tolerated, after a minimum of 2 weeks of treatment, the dose may be increased to 3 mg BID. Subsequent increases to 4.5 mg BID and 6 mg BID should be attempted after a minimum of 2 weeks at the previous dose. Exelon should be taken with meals in divided doses in the morning and evening.

Exelon use is associated with significant stomach-related side effects, including nausea, vomiting, loss of appetite, and weight loss. Inform your doctor of any side effects as these side effects can be serious. Additional information on Exelon can be found on the website www.exelon.com.

Razadyne™ ER (Galantamine HBr)
Razadyne ER is also in the class of drugs called acetylcholinesterase inhibitors and is available in three dosage strengths, 8-mg, 16-mg, and 24-mg extended-release capsules. It is indicated for those with mild to moderate Alzheimer's disease. Razadyne ER has the added benefit of being an extended-release capsule, taken only once a day. The most common side effects are nausea, vomiting, diarrhea, loss of appetite, and weight loss.

More information on Razadyne ER can be found on the website www.razadyne.com.

Namenda® (Memantine HCl) was the first medication approved to treat moderate to severe Alzheimer's disease. Namenda is believed to work by attaching to the NMDA receptors in the brain and regulating the activity of glutamate. (See Chapter 9 for additional information).

Namenda is supplied in the form of a tablet that is taken twice daily. Therapy begins at 5 mg and gradually increases to the target dose of 10 mg twice a day. Namenda is available in 5 and 10 mg tablets, so a combination of tablets is needed to gradually increase therapy. When the daily dose has reached 20 mg (i.e., 10 mg, twice a day), patients taking Namenda can continue with that daily regimen, unless instructed otherwise by their doctor.

Namenda can be used by itself, or in combination (combination therapy) with Aricept (Donepezil).

Side effects are rare but the most common adverse effects reported with Namenda are dizziness, confusion, headache and constipation and other side effects may occur. Inform your doctor of any side effects so that he/she may consider changing dosage or alternative therapies.

More information on Namenda can be found on the website www.namenda.com.

Combination Drug Therapy
Some recent studies have shown that patients may benefit from a

combination of therapies, particularly the combination of Aricept and Namenda. Ask your doctor about these developments, and ask what the best form of therapy is for your loved one.

Treating Other Symptoms Associated with Alzheimer's Disease
Antipsychotics (neuroleptics, tranquilizers) may be helpful if the person with Alzheimer's disease suffers from hallucinations, delusions, or agitation. It has been estimated that about one third of people with Alzheimer's disease are prescribed antipsychotic drugs. However, a recent paper that combined data from various sources has concluded that patients with Alzheimer's disease may have a higher risk of dying than those without Alzheimer's when prescribed antipsychotics. These drugs should be used only under the supervision of a physician.

These medications should not be used if the person is merely annoying you. They are not designed to make the caregiver's life easier, but to help to control abnormal behavior or psychiatric disturbances. They are prescribed for specific usage and you should follow your physician's instructions carefully. Some of the most commonly prescribed behavioral medications to reduce aberrant behavior (violent, repetitive, anxiety, pacing, and obsessive behavior) include Seroquel, Depakote and Resperidone.

Other Therapies
(See also estrogen therapy for women, anti-inflammatory drugs, antioxidants, and antidepressants above.)

Gene Therapy
Genetically modified tissue, designed to boost a naturally occurring protein that stimulates cell function and stops cell death, has been implanted into some patients with Alzheimer's disease. Further studies are needed to determine just how effective this therapy can be.

Exercise
Exercise may be helpful. It can support better cardiovascular health, which may result in better blood flow to the brain so improving brain function. In the later stages of Alzheimer's disease, exercise becomes more important. A person with Alzheimer's will start to

lose strength, flexibility, balance, and endurance and exercise may help to maintain these functions. One study suggests that in women, for every mile walked per week, there was a 13% less chance of dementia. Recent studies have supported the idea that exercise, even if started late in life, can be beneficial in reducing the risk of developing dementia, and may even help slow the progression of the disease in those already afflicted. One study showed that exercising as little as walking for fifteen minutes three times a week is enough to reduce the risk of developing dementia.

Mental Exercise
Individuals that keep mentally alert in their middle years, whether from a mentally demanding occupation or from intellectual hobbies, have been shown less likely to develop Alzheimer's.

Diet, Hydration, and Nutritional Supplements
It is important to encourage the person with Alzheimer's disease to eat well and drink often. They may forget, so try different techniques and be patient, as they will generally take longer to eat.

- o Eat on a regular schedule.
- o Minimize distractions.
- o Offer one kind of food at a time.
- o If the Alzheimer's patient wears dentures, make sure they are not causing pain.
- o Try finger foods.
- o Give a multivitamin daily.

Vitamins may be helpful, as some deficiencies (such as with vitamin B6, B12 and folic acid) can lead to symptoms that resemble cognitive impairment. Studies in animals and humans indicate that diets high in folate (leafy green vegetables, asparagus, broccoli, liver, and many types of beans and peas, as well as fruits such as oranges and bananas, also fortified bread). may help reduce the risk of developing Alzheimer's disease, but it is unclear if there is any benefit after the disease has developed.

It has been shown that older adults may have deficiencies of micronutrients such as zinc and there may be a correlation between low zinc levels and more neuritic plaques in Alzheimer's patients. Consider a zinc supplement.

A recent study indicated that soy and fish oils (containing omega-3 fatty acids and, in particular, an omega-3 fatty acid called DHA – docosahexaenoic acid) may help to protect the brain against the memory loss and cell damage caused by Alzheimer's.

If the individual suffers from insomnia, consider some dietary adjustments, such as reducing caffeine intake (coffee, tea, some sodas, chocolate). Avoid tobacco products. Keep a regular schedule, exercise, and undertake activities during daylight hours to develop a routine and help increase sleeping at night. Sleep medications should be considered a last resort, as overuse of these drugs can cause rebound insomnia, an increase in sleeplessness as a response to the medication, falls, and cognitive impairment.

More Therapies
Some other therapies may be helpful in managing the person with Alzheimer's disease.

Music therapy — Playing light music can be relaxing and provide a more comfortable and enjoyable environment and help to ease stressful situations.

Light therapy — There is some anecdotal evidence that suggests that bright lighting may actually have a positive impact on the mood, behavior, and sleep of adults with dementia. There are clinical trials ongoing. Since there would be few, if any, side effects, this certainly seems worth trying. You might also test the benefits of being out in the sunlight with the Alzheimer's patient.

Pet therapy — There have been many positive experiences where dogs and other furry and feathered animals have been introduced to Alzheimer's patients. The therapeutic benefits to the patients, depending on the patients' level of dementia, include helping them to recall long-term memories, increase communication, and become more mobile and social. If you do not have pets in your family, contact your neighbors or friends to see if they will let you and the person with Alzheimer's spend time together with their pet.

Dolls, Teddy Bears and Robotic Toys — Dolls and teddy bears may help give Alzheimer's patients a sense of ownership and responsibility that they can control, identify and bond with. They may also provide a topic of conversation for the patient that will enable them to interact more with the people in their world. Dolls appear to help alleviate agitation, overcome communication difficulties and reduce withdrawal in some patients and present a low cost therapy that is worth trying.

Robotic Toys may provide an alternative to live pets as a source of comfort and a distraction for the person with Alzheimer's disease. These toys can respond when stroked, make appropriate feedback sounds and have the advantage of not needing care although they tend to be expensive.

7. Tips and Tools for the Caregiver

Many of the topics to be discussed in this chapter have been raised previously in this book. We now want to give you some suggestions on how to manage some of the more serious and more common problems that you will encounter when caring for the person with Alzheimer's disease.

Your relationship with them will change forever as you take over the role of caregiver and relinquish the role of spouse or family member. However, this does not mean that you can no longer enjoy each other's company. If you plan well, organize your lives, take one day at a time, and provide love and care, you will be able to have many more enjoyable times together. Approach the problems with knowledge and patience and learn to respond to the patient's behaviors positively, no matter how extreme they may seem. A sense of humor will not go amiss.

REMEMBER, the patient does not choose to do or say the things they do. These things are a consequence of damage to the brain caused by Alzheimer's. It is important for you to recall this fact when they speak in a hurtful manner. Repeat to yourself, "It's just the disease talking." Also, repeat to yourself, "Let it go. What does it hurt?" or "Who is this behavior hurting?" Your life as a caregiver will be a whole lot easier if you remember to ask yourself these questions. Do not worry about the small stuff; let it go, particularly if they are enjoying themselves. Only intervene if their behavior is harmful to themselves or to others.

The impact of caring for a person with Alzheimer's cannot be underestimated and is perhaps one of the biggest commitments a person can face. However, if approached positively, it can be a commitment filled with hard work and emotional stress that can also be meaningful and rewarding.

The vast majority of caregivers are caring for a parent or spouse and half of all caregivers live in the same residence as the person with Alzheimer's, making theirs a 24-hour-a-day job. Despite the personal and financial sacrifices reported by many caregivers, the vast majority feel their duties are a "labor of love".

Managing Daily Activities

The most important thing that you can do to manage the daily activities for the person with Alzheimer's disease and for you is to establish and follow a daily routine. This will give a sense of security to the patient and will give them something they can look forward to on a daily basis. Also, it will ensure that you make time for yourself. Write out the schedule and put it on the refrigerator to remind you of the activities planned each and every day.

Activities

You may be asking what the person with Alzheimer's disease can or should be doing all day? A good source for activity is a social model day care program for individuals with Alzheimer's, as this is why the service exists. If you are unable to find one or you do not have a program such as this in your area, *you* will become the Activities Director. You will have to build the skills to create successful activities. Activities are important because they focus on the social, cognitive, memory recall and hand-eye coordination abilities of the individual with Alzheimer's. You should build activities that stimulate these abilities, but keep activities short and do not expect too much because the person is impaired and may tire easily. Choose simple activities that you may do concurrently such as games, karaoke, folding the clothes, discussing memories or recent events, talking of friends and family, listening to music the person enjoyed from the past, or taking them for a walk or on an outing. You can also get a balloon and bounce the balloon back and forth, which helps to improve coordination skills and cardiovascular fitness. Try to avoid games like bingo and tic-tac-toe that will be too complex for those with moderate and severe symptoms. Provide adult-appropriate and relevant activities. Activities that make the person feel useful are equally, if not more, important (such as household tasks or gardening). If you do not have this type of activity, create one; for example, take clean towels, unfold them, place them in a basket, and ask the person to fold them or take clean dishes from the cupboard, place them in the sink, and ask the person to wash the dishes. Either way, you must celebrate what they can do, never scold them. Work at their pace. Make sure to help the person get started on the activity by breaking the activity down into easy, clear steps and cue them along the way. You should perform the activities as part of your daily routine. Remember to look for signs of agitation or frustration within the activity and if this occurs, validate the person's feelings and redirect them to something else.

Plan of Care
The physician and the health care team should have provided you with a plan of care that may include prescriptions or other therapies to treat the symptoms of the disease. You, the caregiver, will take responsibility to make sure that the plan of care is followed accurately and you undertake to communicate with the health care team so that you are well informed and so that you understand the treatment and the expectations of the health care plan. You should build the health care plan into the daily routine that you have established for yourself and for the person with Alzheimer's disease. The routine will help to establish a feeling of success and independence for the individual because they can help to take care of themselves. You can offer assistance when they need it or you can cue them so that they can do things for themselves.

Communicating with the Alzheimer's Patient
In order to understand how the person with Alzheimer's disease feels, imagine for a moment that you wake up in a foreign land where nobody speaks English. You do not know what language they are speaking, nor can you read signs or ask for directions. You cannot even find the bathroom and you have no idea about their culture or social values. Can you imagine the frustration of not being able to understand or communicate? Welcome to the world of Alzheimer's!

Losing the ability to communicate effectively is one of the most devastating effects of any disease for the patient. The ability of humans to communicate with highly developed language is one of the features differentiating us from other animals. The loss of this skill has a profound affect on the well being of the patient and can result in frustration and depression. For the Alzheimer's patient, they will eventually lose the ability to communicate by any means — verbal, gestures, touch, or any other.

As caregiver, the way in which you communicate will have to change. The patient will lose the capacity to understand complex language and will be confused easily if what you are saying is not crystal clear. You must try to be patient and not get frustrated with them as this may affect your tone of voice, which may be interpreted by the patient as that you are angry with them or otherwise unhappy with them and this may increase their confusion and agitation. Facial expressions and gestures are just as important as the spoken word and your intonation, so you should be aware of how you may appear to the individual and try to control any negative expressions and gestures.

When speaking with the person, you should avoid speaking to them as if they were a child or a baby, or as if they were not in the room. Nor should you interrupt them while they are speaking. Make sure to say their name before you speak to them and make sure that you have their attention. If you are asking a question, allow enough time for the person to answer. If they cannot communicate their thought and they are searching for a word, gently try to provide them with the word they are seeking.

Validation and Redirection Therapy
The practice of Validation and Redirection therapy has become the universally accepted way of coping with behaviors while properly communicating with someone who is affected by Alzheimer's disease. This is more technique than therapy, as it is up to the caregiver to validate the person's feelings, thoughts, or fears and then redirect them to a more positive activity.

Example: Frank is very upset. He is insisting that strangers have entered his room and taken his favorite shirt. You see that Frank is very agitated. To calm him down, you should approach Frank and ask him if you can help him or ask him what is wrong. Then validate this feeling of violation and reassure Frank by sympathizing with his feelings, be compassionate and assure him that you will find the culprit, and then redirect Frank by asking him to help you with a task he is very good at. It is important that you smile, speak slowly and gently, and be conscious that this feeling is very real to Frank.

Example: Betty is sobbing; she is asking to go home. You should approach her and identify why she is crying, then validate the feeling that she is homesick. As you are validating her feeling, ask her to "tell" you about home, support her feelings (she is looking for security), and then redirect her to a helping activity that she will enjoy.

As the disease progresses, it will become increasingly difficult for the patient to follow a conversation, so again you will have to be patient with them so that you can understand what they are trying to say and what they want. Eventually, they will lose the ability to converse altogether.

Here are a few tips to be able to communicate with your loved one. Remember, communication is both verbal and nonverbal (facial expressions, gestures, body language).

- o Keep it simple; use short, clear sentences.
- o Be very specific, unambiguous.
  - Call them by name, so that they know you are talking to them.
  - Avoid pronouns; if you are talking about someone, use their name and not he or she.
- o Keep questions simple, so that you can get a yes or no answer.
- o If they are having trouble following the conversation, repeat their last words to try to maintain some continuity.
- o Be positive with your conversation and give them positive feedback.
- o Keep your facial expressions and gestures positive. Smile and nod and point toward things to help explain what you are saying.

When communicating, try to keep eye contact and be on the same level; that is, both of you sitting down or both of you standing. If they break off eye contact, this may mean that they have not understood what you are saying, but do not want to admit it. If you lose eye contact or if they turn away or walk away, touch them to let them know that you are there and want to talk to them. Make them feel part of the conversation. Touching should be gentle and reassuring.

Keep aware of their body language. If they are getting upset or anxious, you may be pressing them too hard, so back off and start again or just try again later. Try to get a response from them, either verbal or a simple nod of the head, so that you know they have understood what you want. If you are unable to get a response, try again or come back to it later when they may be more receptive.

Remember to pace yourself at their speed of communication and practice redirection and validation. In order to help ease tensions, fear, or anxiety, it is important that you understand that you may have to be creative at times and use colored truths.

Example: Bob is delusional and says, "The men in the corner are laughing at me!" When you look, you see no men; you two are alone. You say, "Bob, there are no men in the corner!" Bob then becomes very agitated. A better approach to avoid the agitation is for you to say something like, "Bob, I'm so sorry they are laughing at you; that must not feel good. Let's go to the other room and then I will ask them to leave." It is important that you validate a feeling.

Example: Glenda is sitting on the front porch on a hot summer day; she is insisting that her mother is coming to get her. You say, "Glenda, your mother has been dead for 36 years!" Glenda bursts into tears; she has heard for the very first time that her mother is dead. You have caused pain and confusion by telling the truth. Instead you should say, "Glenda, your mother called on the phone and said she is running a bit behind schedule and she has asked me to have you come inside and wait for her because it is very hot." There is nothing wrong with coloring the truth, playing make-believe, if it is more beneficial to your spouse, friend, or sibling rather than confronting them with the real truth. Their reality is not our reality and in their minds, "Mom" is still very much alive. You must ask yourself this question, "Who is it hurting?" This is not wrong, as it benefits the person with Alzheimer's and causes less emotional distress.

As Alzheimer's progresses, the communication skills of the person affected start to degrade and you, as the caregiver, may feel as if you have moved into an alternate reality. In fact, you have, because the person's words and behaviors make no sense to you. Now, thinking about this from their perspective, you will realize that your words may be just as difficult to understand by the person with Alzheimer's. This results in misunderstandings, igniting tempers, increasing agitation, and making communication even more difficult. Your behavior and approach affects both you and the person with Alzheimer's, so try to stay calm and remember that it is incredibly frustrating for both of you.

The person with Alzheimer's cannot remember. Not being able to find words, explain feelings, or describe needs are a constant problem and source of frustration, and it only gets worse over time until the person may eventually not be able to speak, a condition called *aphasia*.

While the person is still able to communicate, they may develop a condition called *echolalia,* where they repeat words over and over or repeat what you have just said, almost like a skipping record. As the brain cells are dying, a person loses their ability to recall immediate and short-term memory and may repeat questions over and over, such as "What time is it?" or "Where are we going again?"

Sometimes, the person may substitute one word for another incorrectly or may just invent an entirely new word for a familiar object because they are unable to recognize it, but they may be able to identify its use. This condition is called *agnosia*. As an example, a person may have difficulty recognizing an object as a cup or identifying a sound as a cough.

People with Alzheimer's may also:

o   Call you names, make hurtful statements, or become angry with you.

o Yell or cry for no reason.
o Be easily distracted or lose their train of thought.
o Struggle to organize words logically.
o Be unable to form full and recognizable sentences.
o Need more time to figure out what you are saying.
o Use offensive language, such as curse words or ethnic slurs.

It is important for you to make allowances for their communication style and remember that they are not acting this way on purpose. They have a disease that is killing their ability to communicate. Also, remember that in caring for them, they are never wrong in their minds. While this may be hard to deal with because you know you are right and they are wrong, you are the caregiver and you must have their best interests at heart. *They are right 100% of the time!*

Do not take it personally — As frustrating as it may get with the person's inability to communicate or if they lash out at you by calling you names, putting you down, or yelling at you, do not take it personally; it is the disease talking, not your loved one.

Use a calm, relaxed tone of voice and smile — If your words and the way you say them do not match, it may be confusing. Your nonverbal cues often send a clearer message than your words. Always approach the person with a smile; we as humans do not just communicate with words, but also with body language. Use a smile when talking with your loved one.

Keep things simple — Use short sentences and plain words. Avoid complicated questions or directions. Ask yes/no questions and cue the person while they are attempting to follow your directions. Do not criticize them.

Do not interrupt — It may take several minutes for your loved one to respond. Avoid criticizing, hurrying, correcting, and arguing.

Validate their feelings — Your loved one may cry, get upset, have outbursts, or display anger or sadness in various ways. Before you get angry, stop to think about their feelings, fears, or frustration. After all, they may realize that something is wrong with them and they cannot remember; everyone is entitled to have a bad day now and again. Validate their feelings, identify why they are upset by asking them how they feel or why they are mad, then comfort them by repeating what they have said, offer understanding, and redirect them to a more positive activity.

Applaud their "good tries" and accomplishments — It is important to help them feel successful and secure.

Show interest, maintain eye contact — Maintain eye contact and stay near them so they will know that you are listening and trying to understand. Make sure to squat down to their eye level if they are sitting because standing above someone can feel threatening.

Use visual and verbal cues to increase recognition — If they have to go to the bathroom, take them to where the toilet is visible. Say, "We're going to use the toilet" and if they are able, cue them on how to unbutton their pants and use the toilet. Or, if you believe they need to use the bathroom and you are unsure if they can understand your question, take them to the bathroom and point to it before asking if they need to go to the bathroom.

Avoid distractions and noise — With a background of sounds or noise, communication can be difficult for anyone; with Alzheimer's, it is almost impossible. The person with Alzheimer's can become overwhelmed by too much noise and distraction. Their brain cannot handle all the information and your conversation may not be heard while they are distracted by the background noise.

Make Your Home a Safe Place
As the patient's cognitive functions decline, their awareness will also decline. They will forget what household items are for or where they belong. Remember also that the patient can become violent. You, as the caregiver, must take a close look at your home and make it as safe as possible for the patient and for you. It is a good idea to ask a friend or family member to look at your house after you have made the initial efforts at safety. There may be things you are comfortable with that others can see that might be potentially damaging or could even be used as a weapon. There are many items

such as childproof locks that can be very helpful to secure your home.

To help the patient move around the home and to find the things that they need, it is important to be consistent. Always put items away in the same place and encourage the patient to do the same. If it becomes necessary, you can label cupboards and rooms with their contents so that the patient can still find them without having to ask and so they can retain some level of independence as long as possible. Put a nameplate on their own room (and yours and the bathroom) so they know where they are. You can have some fun with this by making the nameplates yourselves and creating an activity that you can do together. Of course, this will become increasingly difficult in the later stages of the disease as the patient becomes more dependent on you.

Look for any item that can be dangerous to the patient or can be used as a weapon — knives, tools, medicines, cleaning fluids, and other chemicals such as fertilizers, herbicides, and pesticides. If you keep guns or hunting items in the house, lock them up and put them out of sight.

Wandering is one of the common symptoms of Alzheimer's disease. Not recognizing their own home is another. We do not know why individuals with Alzheimer's wander, but as many as 60% of those with the disease will wander. You do not want the patient to leave the house without your knowledge. It can be dangerous for them and a cause of stress and anxiety for you. Make sure that all doors and windows have locks and chains either positioned high so they cannot be reached easily or are complex to operate with a key or keys. Alarms may be frightening to the patient, but consider using alarms if the patient can tolerate them. Do not forget that you may need to secure some passageways to prevent access (such as at the top of stairs). Childproof gates are generally sufficient for this, but you may need something stronger. Remove area rugs, electrical cords, and any obstructions that they might trip over.

Make sure that your house is well lit during the day and use night-lights at night so that the patient can see clearly when they are moving around. If they have access to a yard (fenced in), make sure that the yard is well lit at night. If you have a swimming pool, put a baby fence around the pool so they cannot fall in.

Glass or mirrored doors can be a hazard. How many of us have walked straight into a patio door because it is so clean we thought that it was open? Put stickers on glass doors so they are clearly visible. The stickers used to stop birds from flying into windows work just fine. You can have some fun with the patient sticking these on or even getting them to make your own to stick on.

Look for things that can get hot (stove, fireplace, matches, curling tongs, toaster, electric frying pan, etc.) and make sure they are either kept out of the way or are disabled (take the knobs off the stove) or protected (fire guard) so the patient cannot turn them on and burn themselves. Hot water can scald. Have the thermostat on your water heater turned down so that you still have hot water, but it is not so hot as to scald.

Bathrooms or any room that can get wet can be a dangerous place for the patient. Make sure that there are grab bars in bathtubs and other necessary locations, and use nonslip matting wherever it may be needed in bathtubs, shower stalls, or on the floor in the bathroom, laundry room, or mud room.

Get your loved one an identity bracelet or necklace with your contact information on it. Alzheimer's patients wander off and while you will do your best not to let them wander out of your sight, sometimes it happens and you want to let people know that your loved one is memory impaired and to contact you immediately so that you can go to collect them.

Much of this seems common sense and indeed it is, but it is something that needs to be done to protect you, the patient, and your home from accidents that can be prevented easily.

Personal Care
The Alzheimer's disease patient will forget or may just become apathetic about their personal hygiene. Depending on the severity of the disease, they may not remember when they last bathed, cleaned their teeth, or changed their clothes. If they can take care of daily

hygiene themselves, encourage them to do so and let them do it to preserve their privacy and dignity, even if it takes them a long time.

Plan personal hygiene tasks into their daily routine and make sure that all the items they will need to use are readily available and in their usual places. Make it so that completing these tasks is not optional, but something that they must do as part of their daily routine.

If the patient needs help, be gentle and prompt when you can. If you have to intervene, take your time and encourage them to try to help themselves, but you can hand them the soap, run the water, lay out their clothes, etc. Try not to give them choices that might confuse them. If a bath or a sponge bath is easier, make the choice for them, but be consistent. If liquid soap is easier than bar soap, make sure that no bar soap is available. Make sure that they are closely supervised when it comes to the more difficult and possibly dangerous tasks such as shaving. Be ready to (gently) take over this function for them or let them know how good they look with a beard and avoid shaving altogether. Take every precaution to be safe.

If you notice changes in personal hygiene habits, if they resist having you help them, or they refuse to participate in personal hygiene activities, look into the reasons for their reluctance. The reasons may be that the shower is too noisy (try a bath) or they may like to wear the same outfit each day. If they are reluctant to bathe, make an effort to ease tension by installing grab bars and a handheld showerhead. Having low running water that you or they can direct may be better than having water pouring from above. Hand them a washcloth and cue them to start washing and help them if needed. They may feel shame or embarrassment, so it is important that you help to ease this feeling. Explain step by step what you are doing and help them to feel in control. Try some soothing music. Reward them with a warm bathrobe and praise them for their efforts. If they simply will not shower or take a bath, try moist towelettes. Avoid power struggles over bath time that may diminish their feeling of independence or pride.

If they want to wear the same outfit every day, you may want to buy several sets of the same clothes, so that soiled clothes can be washed. Try keeping a clean set in the hamper to swap with the dirty outfit, so that they do not notice that you have changed the outfit.

Incontinence

Losing one's ability to control bodily functions creates a feeling of helplessness and embarrassment for any individual, and may be a source of great stress for the caregiver. Realize that incontinence is a symptom of the disease and the ability for the person to remember if they have been to the bathroom is gone. Because they are ashamed of the incontinence, you may find that they may hide their soiled garments or bedding. Remember, this is pride and nobody wants to feel embarrassed. To manage the incontinence, fit a bathroom schedule into the daily routine where you remind them to go to the bathroom every 2 hours or after meals and before bedtime. You can also use physical reminders, such as leading them gently by the hand to the bathroom and by using a pleasant voice, with a smile. Encourage them and do not be bossy or rough. If they need to be changed, play some soft music they enjoy and change their clothes next to the toilet. It is a good idea to use the grab bars installed in the bathroom so they can hold onto the bars as you change them or have a washcloth or other soft item for them to hold onto while they are being changed.

Remain calm, even if the situation becomes difficult. It may be that the person becomes agitated when you want to help change their clothes. If so, walk away and try again in 10 minutes. Always remember to approach with a smile. Never blame or scold them for their accidents. Explain to them, step by step, what you are doing. After all, think about this, would you want someone you do not know coming in, grabbing you, pulling your pants down, and telling you that you soiled yourself?

If you notice that the person's accidents are increasing, you should decrease the toileting schedule from once every 2 hours to once every hour and half, hour, etc. until you can cope with the incontinence effectively. It may be a good idea as well to consider using pull-ups (adult briefs) to help control any bodily contaminants from soiling the carpets, bed, or furniture. When you are changing or cleaning someone after using the bathroom or cleaning up after an accident, you should always wear latex or non-latex gloves, dispose of briefs properly, and wash your hands thoroughly. Moreover, if the person is wearing briefs, you should utilize barrier cream on their skin to reduce any opportunity of rash or skin breakdown. You must also stay vigilant about urinary tract infections (UTIs). UTIs are common in those who are incontinent. Look for signs in changes of behavior such as lethargy and agitation, facial grimacing, or their hands making fists while urinating. A UTI may be the reason for the person's resistance to using the bathroom.

Bathing

Showering or bathing can be a challenge with Alzheimer's disease. The experience can be frightening and confusing for a person with memory impairment. We discussed previously a bit about showering where you learned to cue and encourage the person to bathe themselves, use sponge baths if needed, or use the reproach method if resistance is occurring.

In order to make the experience of bathing more enjoyable or acceptable, take into consideration the person's previous habits throughout their life. (For example, Mary only used a bathtub every other day, whereas Frank took a shower every night before bed.) You should respect that this experience may be frightening or worse, humiliating. Be gentle and respectful and slowly go through what you are doing step by step. Never rush a person with Alzheimer's into a shower, soap them up quickly, and then push them out without a warm robe because this can be shocking and too intense. Be sensitive to water and room temperature, warm up the room, place extra towels around, and test the water temperature before beginning. You should also incorporate the bath routine around the time the person is calm and most agreeable. Prepare in advance by having all bathing supplies ready, the bath drawn, or the shower on.

An additional challenge you may encounter in the bathroom, where there are usually mirrors, is the patient not recognizing their own image in the mirror. They are looking at a complete stranger. They may become confused and agitated. You should turn them away from the mirrors and point them to a new activity and then cover up the mirrors so they do not have to endure the experience again.

Dressing

You may not realize that getting dressed can be quite a complicated activity as a series of challenges are ever present. These challenges include choosing what to wear, getting soiled clothes off, and getting the new clothes on while trying to manipulate buttons or zippers. You learned earlier in the chapter about dressing and keeping outfit choices to a minimum, as well as dealing with resistance to changing clothes or outfits. Now let us discuss this activity further.

When you are dressing the person with Alzheimer's disease, allow them the opportunity to help dress themselves with you standing by to assist if needed. Whether you are helping or they are performing the task themselves, always provide step-by-step cueing. Be clear in your prompting, but allow them the opportunity to help themselves. The longer they can dress themselves, the longer they may be able to retain the skill. If they are able to dress themselves, do not do it for them, and allow enough time as not to rush or place pressure on them. Make this a part of the daily routine at the same time each day. Choose clothing that is comfortable, yet sufficient, to keep the person cool or warm, easy to get on or off, and does not require a lot of struggling with buttons or zippers. Elastic waistbands in underwear and outer clothing can be uncomfortable and cause irritation. Many clothing manufacturers offer soft-banded waistbands that do not have the bunching effect of elastic. If you cannot locate this type of clothing, you can turn the waistband down around the top of the seam so the elastic rests on cloth rather than on the skin.

Oral Hygiene

Brushing teeth, flossing, and routine oral hygiene becomes increasingly difficult for the patient to do alone. For the caregiver, it becomes a bigger problem if the patient is uncooperative and will not allow help. However, it is essential that the caregiver find a way to accomplish this task. Oral bacteria that are normally kept under control in the mouth that is frequently cleaned and maintained with good oral hygiene methods will proliferate if the mouth is neglected.

Under normal circumstances, this will lead to problems with teeth and gums and bad breath, but with the severe Alzheimer's patient who has problems with swallowing and who aspirates their food, the inhalation of food and bacteria-rich saliva into the lungs can lead quickly to pneumonia. Pneumonia is one of the most common causes of death for the person with Alzheimer's disease.

Make teeth cleaning a part of the daily routine. Place their toothbrush and toothpaste in a convenient place so that you can gently point to them if prompting is needed. If the patient is able to floss, let them do it. If they will let you do the flossing, take the opportunity. If flossing becomes impossible, then use alternatives such as the commonly available mouthwashes.

Nutrition and Hydration
Maintaining good nutrition and hydration are challenges you will face while caring for someone with Alzheimer's disease. These challenges present in various ways:

o   Person refuses to eat or drink.
o   A loss of manual dexterity inhibits them from being able to manipulate utensils.
o   Cognitive difficulties make them unable to recognize utensils or edible foods.
o   Gastrointestinal problems.
o   Difficulty with swallowing, which may lead to choking.
o   Does not want to wear dentures.
o   The ability to taste may be impaired.

In addition to these problems, the individual may forget they have eaten, so they eat again, which can lead to an increase in weight, or they may believe they have eaten when they have not or may not desire to eat at all, which may cause weight loss.

The person you are caring for may experience one or several of these difficulties or they may not experience any at all.

Caregivers often ask why the individual they are caring for wants to eat sugary or salty foods. Taste sensation is diminished in the person with Alzheimer's, so stronger flavors and textures are preferred.

Seek and follow the advice of a registered dietician and liven up their food with products such as Mrs. Dash, Splenda, low-sodium soy sauce, hot sauce, etc. Keep a careful watch on their diet. The goal is to get them to eat a balanced diet and to make sure they are properly nourished. Unless the person is morbidly obese or diabetic, there should not be a reason to deny the person an occasional sugary treat.

If the individual is refusing to eat, consult your physician. They may offer to prescribe an appetite stimulant. If the individual eats very little or refuses to eat some things, but not others, concentrate on their likes, not their dislikes. Even if they eat the same type of sandwich for lunch and dinner, it is better than nothing at all. In addition, if all they want to eat is ice cream or they are motivated by sweets, you can buy sugar-free ice cream and blend it with a nutritional supplement drink such as Ensure or Carnation. This helps to sustain nutritional/food intake and maintain their weight while other methods are explored to stimulate their appetite and maintain a balanced diet.

Hydration is very important as the human body depends on water for functioning. Dehydration can cause a myriad of issues, including an increase in lethargy, irritability, memory loss, and a decrease in general mobility. It is key that the individual with Alzheimer's receive hydration in whatever way they can and in a way that they enjoy. Consider low-sodium soup, juices, sports drinks, liquid nutrition drinks, and water. Eight or nine full glasses of water, or equivalent, a day is a good rule of thumb.

As Alzheimer's takes its course, swallowing and chewing problems may occur, which may lead to choking. At the first sign of a swallowing difficulty, contact your physician and ask for a swallowing evaluation as soon as possible. If the person does indeed have an issue, advocate for therapy to teach swallowing strategies and diet modification to keep swallowing safe and efficient.

You can minimize the risk of choking at any stage of the disease by not feeding the individual with Alzheimer's anything that a young child could choke on such as candies (hard, chewy, soft, gum), sausages/hotdogs, snack foods (chips, nuts, crackers), peanut butter, rice (includes sticky), and certain fruits (grapes, cherries, all types of berries). If choking occurs when drinking liquids, a swallowing assessment by a speech language pathologist is recommended. Sometimes, restricting the size of the swallow using a special cup or thickening the liquid using commercially available thickening agents can reduce choking incidents. Thickening agents should be used with caution and only following the advice of the speech language pathologist because the thickening agents are often not well tolerated by the patient and can result in the patient not receiving enough fluids.

Some helpful suggestions to make sure that the person you are caring for eats properly are to:

- o Offer finger foods such as finger sandwiches, cheese wedges, or cut fruit/vegetables.
- o Offer the meals at the same time each day as part of their routine. This will help to establish habit and assist in cueing the person that it is time to eat. As well, schedule small snacks throughout the day.
- o Offer meals wherever the person will eat them, but it is important that you try to establish a routine. This would be even more important in the case of someone who wanders or will not sit at the table.
- o Remember to be patient and allow them, if possible, to feed themselves even if it takes time. Do not rush them, but let them go at their own pace. If you do not, you can risk choking or the person not desiring to eat at all.

Throughout your role as a caregiver, you will meet many challenges. If you remember to always have patience, set a routine, and be proactive for care, your role will be much easier and enjoyable.

Managing Behavioral Problems
We have described many of the behavioral symptoms associated with Alzheimer's disease and here are some tips on how to deal with them. Managing these behavioral problems is without a doubt one of the hardest parts of being a caregiver to the Alzheimer's patient and is frequently the reason that the decision is taken to send

the patient to another facility where they can receive full-time care and relieve the caregiver of the burden. Some of the tips we give may be difficult to implement. It is easy for us to advise, but it is much harder to do. Patience and trying to understand what has caused the behavioral reaction and then finding a solution is the challenge for you. Establishing the daily routine for both of you will help you to create a stable environment that may help to alleviate some of the behavioral problems.

Remember to record each of the behavioral events so that you can discuss them with the health care team the next time you see them.

Environmental Management
We have emphasized the need for consistency and routine for the patient and careful planning on the part of the caregiver so that the patient is confronted with a stable environment they can relate to and feel comfortable in. Any sudden changes (too much noise, too much activity, new furniture) to their environment can trigger behavioral changes in the patient that may manifest in many of the ways described below. You are the one who best knows when or if things in the home might change or if trips are planned, and with the experience you have built up by caring for the patient, you may be able to predict how their behavior may change. By knowing in advance and being prepared, you can help to prevent or minimize some of the behavioral manifestations.

Delusions and Hallucinations
The delusions and hallucinations that are manifest in about 70% of the patients with Alzheimer's disease are very real to the patient and you should not try to dissuade them or argue with them about what they believe is happening (delusions: Who is stealing their money?) or what they are seeing or hearing (hallucinations). Rather, engage them in a conversation about what they believe is happening and gradually redirect the conversation to something that is not stressful to them, such as talking about an item of their daily routine. Be patient and calm. This is not a time to tell them they are crazy or lying to you.

As the disease progresses, and we are now talking probably several years after the initial diagnosis and into the moderate or severe stage, the patient will forget some of the key aspects of their lives. For example, they may forget who you are even though you have lived with them for the last 20, 30, or more years. They will forget where they put things, forget where they live, and may forget what they look like. Forgetting so many things can lead to frustration, anger, and sometimes violence on the part of the patient, much to the distress of the caregiver. The patient tries to find ways to explain these happenings to them and this can result in delusions, hallucinations, and phobias.

Among the most common delusions are the following:

1. They are unable to find things and they cannot remember where they put things, so they believe that people are actually hiding or stealing the items from them. In severe instances of the delusion, they believe that people are actually coming into the house to hide and steal things, and the patient may actually talk to the (imaginary) intruders.

2. They forget that the place in which they are living is their home. They will request to be taken home when they are already there because they do not remember or recognize their surroundings. They may pack bags in order to be taken home. They may actually try to leave the house to find their way home. It is important to note that when someone with Alzheimer's is stating that they want to go home, they are making a statement of feeling. This individual is looking for a feeling of safety and security, in other words, home. "Home" is a place inside that they can never find; it is a feeling. The caregiver can help to explore that feeling by asking, "Could you tell me about your home?" You are validating their feeling and offering security through compassion and interest. These situations are difficult for the caregiver because the patient may be persistent and occasionally violent in their efforts to "go home." Be reassuring and let them know that you are taking care of them and that everything will be all right if they stay with you. Do an activity with them or go for a walk. They are looking for security and safety, not home. Home is a place inside that represents the security you are offering them.

3. What do you do when your spouse no longer recognizes you? They may not know who you are and when you explain it to

them, they may conclude that you are an imposter. This type of delusional behavior can be very upsetting for you who have altered your life to take care of this person that you have loved for many years and now you are not even recognized. Alzheimer's can be a cruel disease in this way, but remember: It is the disease that is responsible and not anything the patient can do anything about. In this case, although it is very difficult, do not confront them and say "I am your wife" because they may only remember you in your 30s, not your 70s. It is better for you to agree and validate their feeling, inject some humor if you can, and give them a hug. Do not argue, even if this hurts. It is better to hug and redirect them to some photos, reminisce, or find another activity.

4. In some cases, the individual with Alzheimer's may experience hallucinations that manifest themselves when the patient believes that they see intruders, dead friends, or relatives and sometimes even smells odors such as fire or hears noises down the hall or disruptions outside. These hallucinations may raise the anxiety level of the patient and the caregiver's role is to calm them and to redirect them to more restful thoughts. Validate the feeling of insecurity, the delusion, or hallucination and then address the figment people by talking directly to them and asking them to leave. This technique will work most of the time.

Agitation and Anger
The patient can become agitated or give angry outbursts because they are frustrated or are confused about what is going on around them. They may have feelings of inadequacy, insecurity, or are simply overwhelmed with what they are doing or cannot deal with too much sensory input (too much noise, too many people talking). Do not try to reason or argue with them about why they are frustrated or why they had an outburst because they will have no answer for you and this may frustrate them even more. Try to be supportive, reassuring, and understanding. Let them know that you are there to help them and solve the problem, and then try taking them to a different setting and redirect the conversation so they can forget the incident.

What do you do if the anger is directed at you? You should consider your situation and your safety. If you feel in danger, get assistance. If you feel they may hurt themselves and you cannot cope alone (maybe they are too big for you to handle), get assistance and finally remove the patient from the environment that made them angry in the first place, and take them to a more relaxing environment.

Profanity
Explicit language and profanity are common occurrences with the Alzheimer's patient. Their memory of what is socially acceptable has deteriorated and they have little or no comprehension of the impact of what they are saying. They may even enjoy the reaction of astonishment that they get from their utterances. With family members and friends, this should not pose too much of a problem as they will already know their loved one is ill and not responsible for their words. Most of what is said can be heard commonly on the television, in movies, and on the playground, so most people will not be too offended. Children can be taken out of the room if necessary. If the patient's profane language becomes a serious problem, you should consider not taking them out in public. Of course, if they are in a health care facility, they will be surrounded by other patients who also will not care.

Inappropriate Sexual Behavior
This is one of the most embarrassing and difficult situations for the caregiver to deal with, but you will have to learn what to do when the patient exhibits inappropriate sexual behavior or makes overt sexual comments. They may decide to undress in public because they are too hot. They may start masturbating or touch other people inappropriately or do other socially unacceptable acts that just feel good to them. They have forgotten or lost the knowledge of appropriate sexual behavior.

In this case, preventive action can go a long way. Give them clothes that are difficult to take off, clothes without zippers, or hold them by the hand so they cannot touch others. If your preventive actions fail, then take them to a private place and try to redirect them to other thoughts or actions.

Equally embarrassing to the caregiver is the sudden outburst of (sexually) explicit comments in public places. They may see a nice looking lady or man with attractive features and inappropriately blurt out sexual comments in a public place, another unfortunate consequence of the disease. These behaviors can be associated with a general loss of inhibitions or a general lack of judgment in the person with Alzheimer's disease, or the loss of inhibitions may simply make them more sexually interested.

Some of the acts that may be exhibited include:

o Hypersexuality.
o Aggressiveness that is inconsistent with past sexual behaviors.
o Forgetting social/sexual graces (sexual manners).
o Reacting overtly to what feels good; mistaking personal care as being sexual.
o Forgetting the steps to having sex (*apraxia*); having more abrupt approaches to sex.
o Misinterprets siblings as sexual partner; self-centered sexual interest.
o Difficulty focusing attention on sex; social withdrawal.
o Decreased interest in sex.

Wandering and Pacing
These are very common symptoms of the person with Alzheimer's disease. If they are restless, bored, feel lost, agitated, or any other reason, they may start to wander or pace. Their wandering can be dangerous to them and they can get lost. When you see them wandering, try to head them off gently so that you can redirect them to a different activity. It is a good idea to let your neighbors know that there is a person with Alzheimer's in the neighborhood so that they can call you if they see the patient wandering off. Make sure that they are wearing their identity bracelet with your contact information engraved on it. When you collect them, talk to them about where they were going. Do not scold them for wandering off.

The Alzheimer's Association has developed a program called "Safe Return". This program is "a nationwide identification, support and enrollment program that provides assistance when a person with

Alzheimer's or a related dementia wanders and becomes lost locally or far from home." More details can be found on the Safe Return website at http://www.alz.org/Services/SafeReturn.asp. We recommend you look into this program and see if it is appropriate for you.

Clinging and Following
When the patient gets disoriented, does not know where they are, or is confused by their surroundings, they may start to follow you around or cling to you. They are probably afraid that you are going to leave them alone in their very confused world. While this can be very annoying to you, try to find a way to distract them and make them feel more comfortable in their surroundings. Finding activities for them to do to distract them from their fears and occupy their minds with a new challenge is a good way to manage the problem so you can get on with what you were doing. You are their safety/security blanket.

Agnosia
As the disease progresses, the patient will have increasing difficulty recognizing familiar people and things. This is called *agnosia*. This may cause confusion, agitation, anger, or some of the other manifestations mentioned. The patient will be better managed if they have a set routine and activities so they can be more easily redirected.

Repetitive Behaviors
You may find that this is a constant issue. It may drive you crazy when the person scrubs one glass for half an hour or asks you repeatedly what time it is. You may feel that they are doing this on purpose (remember the children's game?). They are not. This is an example of short-term or immediate memory loss that is a symptom of Alzheimer's disease and the person has lost their ability to retain information. This means that the person may verbally repeat the same question over and over due to the memory loss. Be patient, reassure them, and answer their question and redirect, because it is better than showing annoyance and creating a larger behavioral issue. To reduce repetitive behavior, use simple, short instructions. Do not ask them to do something for you. For instance, hand them a towel and say, "Would you wipe the counters?" rather than saying,

"Help me with this." Using a nondescriptive statement will only confuse. Simple tasks for someone with Alzheimer's often can be complex. Remember to smile, have patience, ignore mistakes, and praise, praise, praise their accomplishments.

Sleeping Issues

Sleeping patterns may become an issue as the disease progresses. They may stay up at night and sleep during the day. This can be a great stress for you as it can be physically and mentally draining. Sleep is as important as food or water. You can reduce disturbances in sleep patterns by carefully planning the daily routine with exercise periods, chores, and activities so they do not sleep during the day. Walking 30 minutes or more a day may help them sleep better. Also, there is some evidence that increasing the amount of daylight they receive by an hour or more a day, either by being outside or using a light box, may help improve their sleep patterns. Do not allow them to sit and vegetate, they surely will sleep. In addition, caffeine should absolutely be avoided in the person with Alzheimer's disease because caffeine tends to activate the person and increase sleep disturbances and can contribute to behavioral issues.

They also may experience some sleep disturbances due to nightmares. Nightmares can be caused by medications, so try to give the patient their prescription in the morning hours. As well, allow them to sleep wherever they are comfortable, even if it is a chair, couch, or floor. Be sure to make the sleeping area comfortable for them. In order to reduce the amount of disturbance, set bedtime at the same time every night as part of your daily routine; keep the lights dim in the evenings; eliminate loud noise, such as the television; play soft, soothing music; and use night-lights to illuminate the room, hallway, and bathroom.

Aggression

The person with Alzheimer's disease can become agitated easily. They can strike out, fight, throw things, or lash out verbally. If this occurs, they may be telling you that they are scared, hurt, need help, or they do not feel well, but they cannot verbalize it. If this occurs, look for early signs like facial grimacing, body posture, fidgeting, or lack of appetite. Handle the person in a calm reassuring way; do not fight back. Validate their feeling and redirect them to an activity. For example, if they get angry because they cannot zip a zipper, give them a pair of slacks that has a waistband and no zipper. Then praise them for their successful efforts.

What Do You Do When They Resist?

One of the most difficult challenges that you will face is resistance. They may refuse to change their clothes, get out of bed, take a shower, eat, or brush their teeth. This can be particularly frustrating for you as the caregiver. You may not understand why they do not want to do what you want them to do, or why they do not want to take care of their basic needs. You may feel they are doing it on purpose or you may take it personally ("Why are they doing this to me?").

So how do you manage these situations? The first thing you must do is to take a step back, think about your plan of action, and keep your emotions in check. There are many reasons why they may be resisting you, but you must remember that they are sick and it is not personal (they may not even know who you are). When you speak to them, choose your words carefully to relax them and not make them resist you further. You will probably not be aware of the reason for the resistance, but some of the possibilities are:

o Your approach.
o Their general mood or condition.
o Time of day (that is, sundown).
o Effects of medications.
o They are unable to communicate effectively with you.
o Environmental factors may be causing them to be agitated or uncomfortable.
o Over stimulation.
o Depression.

Your frustrations can contribute to their agitation. Take a moment and put yourself in their shoes. As we mentioned earlier, imagine for a moment that you are sitting in your room and someone that you do not recognize suddenly comes into the room, grabs at your arm, says, "Let's go Frank, let's go, let's take a shower," and then begins to take your clothes off. What would you do? Certainly you would consider swatting at the person or resisting their advances. So it is important for you to think before you react to their resistance.

Consider this: Who is it hurting if they do not want to take a shower at 8 a.m. or if they do not want to bathe every day or if they do not want to change their clothes every day? In fact, it is not necessarily good for an older person to bathe every day because their skin may dry out (remember to use a lotion on their skin if it is too dry). It is okay to have the person bathe three times a week. It is not necessary to change clothes every day if they are not dirty or soiled.

As a caregiver, your job is part detective because you may need to find the cause of the resistance. Try to recall the person's previous habits and react accordingly; they may not like to shower in the morning, maybe they showered only in the evening, or they do not like hot showers, but warm showers. Be courteous, be kind, and no matter how frustrating the situation, remember that your behavior is what can be controlled, not that of the person with Alzheimer's.

Always keep in mind that routine will help to reduce the problem of resistance. Plan to schedule the activities of daily living at the same time each day (or, if they are not daily activities, make them the same time each week) and create the routine.

Refusing to Participate
Other situations that may arise are refusal to participate in family or group activities. Environmental factors such as lighting, noise, and large gatherings can overload the brain's already-damaged circuitry. If, for example, there is a group of friends gathering in your home, there may be an individual who is abrasive to the person you are caring for. After all, a person with Alzheimer's disease is still a person and, as people, sometimes we find other people that we do not care for. The person with Alzheimer's is still entitled to that feeling and they may act out or withdraw to tell you they are uncomfortable. Also, loud noises and a lot of activity may cause the person distress and make them tell you once again, "I want to go and I don't like it here."

If the person is depressed, they may withdraw and not want to go anywhere or participate in activities that once brought pleasure. If you are facing this situation, address this with your family physician and ask for a depression workup. If they are diagnosed with depression, you should ask the physician for antidepressant medication. It is your job to help motivate the person to feel better; make sure that you encourage them to participate in an activity or go out for an activity. You must build their self-esteem. With Alzheimer's, particularly for the person who is in the early stage, depression is present as a comorbid condition. This could be caused by shame or embarrassment that they have a problem.

Not Wanting to Move

If a person refuses to move from a chair or get out of bed, they maybe suffering from fatigue as a result of lack of sleep, they may be depressed, or they could be communicating with you that they are in some kind of pain. Pain can be a powerful force, even if the pain is from something as small as an ingrown toenail to a toothache. Ask questions and give them a good look over. If you find something amiss, you should consult your physician and relate your findings.

Refusal to Go to the Doctor or Day Care

When the person with Alzheimer's disease refuses to go to the doctor or day care, you can take steps to counteract their resistance. In this situation, their resistance has to be overcome because these activities are not optional for them.

If you know that you are going to meet resistance, take time out before you get ready to broach the subject of leaving home. Look for a "hook" to get the person out of the house for the appointment. For example, Bob may like chocolate ice cream. If so, then you should incorporate getting some ice cream on your way to or from the appointment. If they are saying that they will not like going, try gaining buy-in with a "try it and see" approach, but do not try to push it. If you push too hard, you may meet more resistance. Additionally, you should give a convincing reason for leaving home. For example, if you are taking them to day care, tell them that their friends are waiting for them and they know they are coming to visit and spend time for the day. If the person is frightened, reassure them, validate their feelings, and let them know that you will be back later to pick them up. Most of all, celebrate what they have done, give positive reinforcement for getting out to day care or going to the doctor, and reward them with your smile and love.

When someone resists, remember to take a step back, think about your approach, assess the situation, make a game plan, and then approach with a smile, asking the person for their help and cooperation.

Managing Other Problems
Driving
Being able to drive a car is widespread and, in many areas, essential just to be able to get around. Most adults know how to drive and probably have driven for many years. The convenience of the automobile to get from one place to another quickly is undeniable and therein lies the problem for the patient with Alzheimer's disease. They know how to drive, have a driver's license, and want to go somewhere, so the natural thing for them to do is take the car.

Now let us take a look at the symptoms of the person diagnosed with Alzheimer's, even in the mild stage. They have some memory loss, they become confused, have a shortened attention span, and decreased ability to calculate. You have to ask yourself, "Is this the kind of person I want driving a vehicle capable of high speed, is highly maneuverable, and weighs thousands of pounds?" The answer should be clearly – NO!

We can make up all kinds of reasons why we think the patient (especially those with the mild form of the disease) can drive, but the reality is that they are unsafe and should be prevented from driving both for their own protection and the protection of others.

The hard part is preventing them from driving. They will be in denial about their condition and will be convinced that they are perfectly capable of driving because they have been doing it for years. It is quite likely that they will not listen to you and it may be very difficult for you to prevent them from getting into the car and driving off. There are a number of things you can do, such as hiding the car keys, telling them the car cannot be driven because the brakes need attention (or some such reason/lie), or telling them that they are no longer insured. These ways may work, however, we suggest that you enlist the help of your doctor. The patient will respect the doctor and their opinions, and will be more likely to believe what he/she has to say. Call ahead to your doctor and let them know you are coming in with the patient and exactly what your problem is so they can be prepared with what to tell the patient. Many doctors are well experienced in managing this situation and will be very happy to help.

In many states, the diagnosis of dementia or Alzheimer's precludes someone from driving and their license will be revoked. Usually, it is the family physician that makes the reports to the appropriate state department.

Holidays or Family Get-Togethers
Holidays and family events are joyous times, but can be bittersweet at the same time. The memories of the person you love with Alzheimer's disease before they were affected may come flooding in, as you recognize the contrast between the person as they are today compared to the way they were. Remember to enjoy the moments and reminisce about the past, but keep in mind this may be an overwhelming experience for the person with Alzheimer's. Establish a balance between rest and activity. Be sure to include the individual in your family traditions, but you may need to adapt to their individual needs and have realistic expectations, as things are different today. If you are celebrating, avoid crowds, changes in routine, and strange surroundings as this may cause confusion and lead to agitation. If you are celebrating in your own home, schedule times for people to visit and keep the crowd to small sizes of one to three people because too many people talking, too much activity, and too much stimulus at the same time can cause behavioral issues. Allow periods of rest and reassure the person you are caring for that they are surrounded by those who love them. It may be helpful when people are saying hello to cue the person with Alzheimer's of their name and who they are within the family. Most of all, make sure to take a few moments out for yourself to enjoy the holiday or event.

Traveling
You will have to make a judgment call on the individual's ability to travel. You will be the one most familiar with their overall health and behavior, and you should take these into account when making your decision.

Traveling with the patient can be rewarding for both of you, but you should plan carefully for any travel and take into consideration what the patient is able to do with their remaining abilities. If travel is a normal part of your routine, so much the better. If it is not, or if a big trip is being planned, the patient may need extra care and attention as you are taking them out of their normal environment. Plan for every eventuality and try to keep the patient's routine (meal times, bedtime, etc.) as normal as possible.

Hospitalization
At some point during the time you are caring for the person with Alzheimer's disease, you may visit the hospital or emergency room. If this happens, you need to make sure that the facility understands that the person has a type of dementia and is unable to make their own decisions. You should already have all of the needed paperwork (such as power of attorney and do not resuscitate orders) in a file in case you do need to go to the hospital. Because of new HIPAA (Health Insurance Portability and Accountability Act of 1996 – patient privacy laws) regulations, you must demonstrate that you are the power of attorney for the incapacitated person. During hospitalization, be aware that the facility may restrain the individual in their bed or provide heavy sedation to calm the person. This is not to be cruel, but to keep the person safe from wandering or falling, and it is for their safety. If the person is not at risk for wandering, there should be no need for restraint.

Many nurses, doctors, and nursing assistants do not understand the nature of Alzheimer's, therefore, you must be the consummate advocate for the individual and do not be afraid to speak up about care. Most importantly, what you must remember is that if a person is on a cholinesterase inhibitor, they should not be taken off of it for any reason unless it interferes with surgical intervention or the person's bodily system is not agreeing with the medication. Many studies have shown that when a person is taken off a cholinesterase inhibitor, they decline and do not ever recover to where they were before the abrupt removal of the medication. Therefore, make sure the hospital gives the person that medication.

After a severe illness or surgery, you may see a significant decline in the person's abilities. This is common in individuals with Alzheimer's. Generally, after long hospitalization due to the aforementioned reasons, the person does not return to the same functional level where they were before the hospitalization.

Long hospitalizations or stays in rehabilitation or skilled nursing homes may cause the person to be bedridden for some time. If this is the case, physical therapy (PT) is needed. Physical therapists often will not complete therapy because the person "cannot remember" the instructions. If this happens, seek facilities that are helpful in locating a private/pay physical therapist who works with geriatric patients.

Moving to Residential Care/Assisted Living
At some point, 5 years after diagnosis on average, you may make the decision to move your loved one to a facility where they can be taken care of on a day-care or full-time basis.

Caregivers often ask, "When is the right time to move the person to residential care?" There is no universal guideline other than that the time is right when you, the caregiver, feel overwhelmed, exhausted, or generally unable to handle caregiving any longer. You may feel some guilt when you make your decision, but bear in mind that what is best for your health is also better for the health of the person for whom you are caring.

Planning for this eventuality will help to ease the problems for both patient and caregiver. Remember, it is you that is making the decision to move them, not their choice for themselves, so the move has to be handled delicately. Whatever your reasons for wanting to move the patient to some form of care, it is important that you do your homework first and make the right decisions.

Start by evaluating why you think the time is right to make the move. Probably, you will have been thinking about this for quite some time and may have discussed it with family and some of your friends. It is useful to get their input and support for your eventual decision.

You should learn what your options are in the types of facilities available in your area. We give some information in this book that will help to guide you, but you will have to do more research for yourself. Talk to your doctor, Alzheimer's Association, and other support groups and go to visit the facilities that have the capabilities to care for your loved one. This will help you come to a decision or at least create a short list of the facilities that are most appropriate for the patient and ones that you can afford. In our opinion, the best choice of care for the person with Alzheimer's disease is a facility that specializes in Alzheimer's care and is a social model program that focuses on quality of life for the resident, rather than just providing them with three meals and a bed. Social model programs are designed to help the cognitive, social, and physical needs of the person with Alzheimer's and concentrate on improving overall quality of life for the individual while giving them a sense of purpose and community. Choose a facility with all-day activities, not just a few activities each day. Continuous social interaction stimulates the brain.

There are many questions that you should ask when you visit the facilities:

- Is there sufficient care or nursing staff? Look at the staff to patient ratio (this should be six or fewer residents to one caregiver).
- What are the qualifications of the nursing staff (do they have experience with Alzheimer's patients)?
- Are they awake and on duty 24 hours a day?
- What is the staff turnover? Is this a stable facility?
- Is this a social model program?
- What medical care is available?
- Do they have a medical director who specializes in Alzheimer's disease?
- Can your doctor visit the facility?
- What activities are available for participation?
- What is the makeup of the patient population?

- o Is it clean, well-maintained, comfortable, calm? Check the facility and environment.
- o What is their policy on restraining patients physically or chemically?
- o Do they have a behavioral management program that does not use behavioral medications except as a last resort?
- o How much privacy will they have?
- o Can they wander around safely?
- o Do they have a secured perimeter?
- o Can residents access the outdoors freely?
- o What training is provided to staff and how much time is spent on training?
- o What is the food like, food options?
- o What is the absolute cost including all extras, points, or levels of care?

Ask to see the last state survey for the facility. Obtain a list of current and past clients that you can call to discuss their experiences with the facility.

As you are making the choice for a facility, you should keep in mind that the facilities are usually run by companies that are in business to make money. You should find a facility that focuses on Alzheimer's care, rather than just on the bottom-line profit. As you seek cost estimates, you should be aware that these facilities utilize three systems of charging for services. They use either an inclusive price program or a point or level system of pricing. Inclusive pricing means that all services are included in one price and you pay by the room size. Points and level systems use a tiered pricing schedule that charges a minimum daily rate, with a special care charge, and then points or levels based on the person's needs. Be wary of the points and level systems because prices can increase dramatically. Inclusive pricing is more reasonable and acceptable for someone with Alzheimer's, as their needs change almost daily. Beware of buy-in fees or community fees, as these fees are generally 30 days of rent up to 60 days of rent that is nonrefundable and charged when moving into the facility. A true care facility will charge a reasonable assessment fee rather than a community fee ($250–$750).

When you have drawn up a short list of facilities or made a selection, you must decide if you will take the patient to view the facility with you. This is a very individual decision that you must make, taking into account how you feel the patient will react. It is a good idea to talk to the support groups and directly with those families that have already made their decisions and can give you the benefit of their experiences to help you make your decision.

Whether or not you decide to show the facility to your loved one, eventually you will make your choice of which facility best suits their needs. Now it is important for you to prepare them for the event, bearing in mind that they may have forgotten that you took them to see the facility, if you did. You must decide on the most appropriate time to tell them about the move. Choose your moment when they seem more capable of understanding and are not agitated or distracted. Prepare what you are going to say and make sure your family and others that the patient meets frequently know the reasons for making the move. The patient will be more comforted if they hear a consistent story. You must decide if you will tell the truth or a partial truth to ease the concerns of the patient. You should anticipate an angry reaction or resistance to the move. If this happens, be prepared to listen and comfort and reinforce what you have already told them so they can get used to the idea of moving. If you decide not to talk to them ahead of moving, be prepared with an answer if they ask. Again, talk to people who have gone through this experience and learn what others have said and what has worked and what has not worked. Digest all this information and apply it to what you know about your loved one and their anticipated reaction.

Once the decision is made on a facility, you can plan the move to make it is as easy as possible for the patient. Talk to the staff at the facility and find out what works best in their experience. If you can distract them and have their belongings in place in their "new home," this may help them to adjust quickly. At least they will be in familiar surroundings with their own possessions in place.

Arrange to visit regularly, so you can stay in close touch with them and monitor how they are being cared for. Take whatever action is necessary if you are not satisfied with the quality of care.

End of Life issues – The Cocoon Theory
The cocoon theory has been proposed by Dr. Patrick Gillette based on end-of-life situations he has observed in many patients. The essentials are reproduced here with his permission.

"We are aware of the concept of 'personal space'. This is known to vary from person to person. For example, people from Wyoming have a large personal space, whereas people from New York City have a small personal space. What I have observed, is that people with dementia convert this concept into the limits of their "world" or a "cocoon". Within this cocoon, they feel safe, secure and peaceful. As the disease progresses, this cocoon begins to shrink. Eventually this becomes more noticeable. One of the hallmarks is walking. People with dementia often stop walking for no apparent reason. There is no physiologic explanation for this, yet, they stop walking. As the disease progresses and the cocoon shrinks further, they no longer are concerned with bladder or bowel control. Hygiene becomes a problem, especially if the caregivers/aides approach the person in a way that disrupts the cocoon. I recommend that they perform hygiene by lifting up the bedding from the bottom, rather than pulling down the bedding, thus preserving the cocoon.

Again, as the disease progresses, they eventually will no longer be interested, or require food and liquids, yet they are at peace within their cocoon. This is often a difficult time for the family/caregivers. The focus should be on the comfort and needs of the person with the dementia. I feel that many of the behavior problems arise from our not recognizing what the person with the dementia needs versus what the family/caregiver thinks they need. As a result the person uses their defenses to try and preserve their cocoon. When everyone realizes that the person is in the terminal phase, the goal should be to maintain dignity and the safety and security of the cocoon. Most patients die from sepsis, but in my practice 'Failure to thrive' is another cause. There are benefits to dehydration, reduced pain, reduced urine output (which reduces the need to change linens and disturbing the person), reduced oral secretions, etc. This does not mean that fluids should not be offered, just careful observation as to what the person wants. This is how we can help preserve the "cocoon" along with the safety, security and peacefulness it offers."

Taking Care of Yourself

You, as the caregiver, have decided to change your life to look after your spouse, family member, or friend who has had the misfortune to develop Alzheimer's disease. If you have followed our suggestions, you will have done your homework, you will have made your plans, and you will have an idea of what to expect in the future. By now, you may have direct experience of how the person in your care is behaving under the influence of the disease. One thing you will know for certain is that the patient is ill and nothing that they say or do is meant to be directed at you; it is simply a consequence of the disease.

Your job as a caregiver to the Alzheimer's patient is demanding, both mentally and physically. Like any other task that requires mental and physical effort, you will be able to cope much better if you are physically and mentally fit and prepared for the task. If you are well prepared, you will be able to handle the most difficult behavior problems (including angry, aggressive behavior) with a confidence that will benefit both you and the person you are caring for.

So what does this mean for you? What are we talking about — mentally and physically fit? First and foremost, it means that while planning your daily routine with your loved one, be sure to make time for yourself. As difficult as this may be in practice, it is important for you and your patient that you do this so that you can recuperate and prepare yourself mentally and physically. It means taking care of *you* with proper diet, exercise, and mental preparation. We will discuss this further in a short while, but before we do, let us take a look at some of the most common statistics related to the well being of caregivers when compared to people that are not caregivers:

- o Caregivers go to their doctor for their own problems almost 50% more often than non-caregivers.
- o They receive over 70% more prescribed medicines than non-caregivers.
- o They suffer more from the effects of stress, including high blood pressure.

   o   They suffer emotional problems that include hopelessness, guilt, anger, despair, and depression.

When you consider what the caregiver has to deal with, especially with the moderate to severe Alzheimer's patient, this is understandable. Treating the symptoms of some of these problems is possible with medication and involvement with support groups where problems can be shared. You will be better able to manage these problems if you are well prepared for them. You will become one of these statistics if you do not take care of yourself.

In many instances, the decision on who the caregiver will be is made consciously. In other words, you choose to take on the task for whatever reason — for love, because you are the best qualified, because you are in the best situation, etc. Having made this choice, and knowing what responsibility you have undertaken, you should accept that it is your choice and prepare yourself to be successful at the tasks in hand. The tasks include not only the care of the patient, but also taking care of yourself.

In other instances, you have become the caregiver by default. Nobody else would step forward to take it on and you are the spouse or closest family member and, therefore, you were landed with the job. In this situation, it is perfectly understandable that you may be angry or bitter at other family members for not stepping forward and this feeling may recur frequently as you deal with the problems of caregiving. However, it is important for your own well being that you put these feelings behind you. You are the caregiver. Follow our advice and plan well. Involve the family members who are willing to help, even though they cannot become the primary caregiver. Find out who are the friends (yours and the patient's) that you can rely on.

As we have suggested, mental and physical fitness will help you to handle these problems. Plan activities for you in your daily routine. You still have a primary responsibility to take care of your loved one, so plan your own activities at a time when you are able to step away from caring for a while — when they are sleeping, when they can be with a friend or other family member, or when they are involved in their activities that do not include you. If you make the effort, you can find time for yourself.

Be aware of what your needs are — You may benefit from talking to your doctor about this. If you have medical problems, you will have to manage these. Take care of your dietary and nutritional needs. Make sure you eat healthily and well. Find out what is a good diet for you by talking to your doctor or nutritionist or consult books and websites. A healthy, well-balanced diet will help to give you the energy you need to take care of the patient and yourself. If you enjoy a glass of wine or other alcoholic beverage, you should continue to enjoy it, but alcohol in excess is damaging to your own health and will impair your ability to take care of your loved one. Smoking and so-called social drugs should be avoided as being detrimental to your health.

Exercise is also important for you — Consult your physician as to what exercise is possible for you and build exercise into your daily schedule. Walking or more strenuous exercise will help to tone your body, keep you reasonably fit, and will help to clear your mind. Exercise with a friend to give you an opportunity to get away from caregiving for a while.

Find time for your own activities — Activities may include hobbies, going to support groups, or visiting family members. Some of these activities can be enjoyed together with the patient, such as listening to music or painting or maybe you enjoy reading to the patient. The important point is that it is time for you and if the patient interferes with your time, the objective is defeated, so look for something you can do without the patient.

We stress it again — *find time for you*. It is too easy to say there is no time. If you are determined and get the help of family and friends, you will find the time. You will benefit and so will your patient.

Helping Children Cope
It is likely that the person with Alzheimer's disease is close to younger people in the family whether they are children, grandchildren, nieces, nephews, or children of friends. Children

will, of course, recognize that there is something wrong with the loved one and they may be among the first to notice something wrong. Children are very perceptive and very aware of changes. Grandpa keeps losing his keys or cannot remember my name or cannot find the words or he seems distant. Children will notice. They are curious and will want to know what is happening to grandpa. Take notice when children tell you something they may have seen or heard. It may be a warning sign.

Give the children as much information as they can understand, depending on their age. Let them know that the loved one is sick and is going to get more sick and may not be as much fun any more. Tell them as much about Alzheimer's as you think they can understand. Give them the information and let them ask questions so you can prepare them in advance for what to expect as the patient deteriorates. By talking to them and showing them books and leaflets that can be obtained from the various support groups, pharmaceutical companies, and websites, you will involve them and help them to manage their relationship with the person with Alzheimer's. Let them explore the books and websites themselves to satisfy their curiosity. Let them know that they have nothing to fear from grandpa, they will not contract grandpa's sickness, and let them understand that just because we will be spending a lot of time looking after grandpa, there will still be lots of time for them.

It is possible that a child is so close to the patient that they exhibit symptoms themselves that can include nightmares, guilt, or depression. If any of these symptoms arise and seem severe to you, you should seek professional help for the child.

Coping with Your Own Anger, Guilt, and Resentment
Our bonds with people are developed over time by shared experiences. Feelings develop because of these past experiences and interactions that can influence our attitudes, perceptions, responses, and reactions.

As you get caught up in the day-to-day stress of caregiving, it is hard for you to step back and be objective and recognize that what the person is doing is not a choice, but the consequence of a debilitating disease. It is so difficult for you to comprehend the unusual actions of the individual that you are caring for. You may find that annoying, negative, or hurtful personality traits are exasperating to you, resulting in anger or resentment toward the person with Alzheimer's disease. Other times, you may find yourself in denial of the seriousness of the situation.

When caregivers feel anger, regret, or resentment in reaction to the difficulty of caregiving, it is normal to experience these emotions. But, this can also be a sign of something more serious such as caregiver burnout. Many times, you will find that your reactions to the patient's behavior are out of proportion to the actual set of circumstances or situation. Your reactions may be attributed not only to the stress of caregiving, but to unresolved feelings of the past or you may not be aware of the underlying cause. Guilt will often creep up and overwhelm you with a feeling of frustration and you may direct your feelings at the person you are caring for. Feelings of anger, guilt, or frustration are counterproductive and expressing these feelings to the person with Alzheimer's is the worst thing you can do, as it will only trigger the behavior that frustrates or angers you.

Behaviors will fluctuate in this disease and the person with Alzheimer's will lose control of their abilities gradually, and due to the disease, the person cannot cognitively accept that the things they do are wrong. It is best for you to take time out, calm down, assess and validate your feelings, and then redirect the person to a more positive activity that you both can enjoy. If you feel unable to cope with the abnormal behaviors, it may be best for you to seek help from a support group or arrange for day care and/or respite services. The only way to beat this terrible disease is to let go of your unreasonable expectations, stop reacting, and educate yourself about the disease. Remember, you have no control of the disease or the person with the disease, you only have control of yourself, and you know stress and frustration are part of the burden of being a caregiver.

Keep the good times in mind, relish the joyful moments, praise yourself for your good work, reward yourself, and reward the person you are caring for with love and affection. This will make it easier to get through difficult days.

When You Need More Help
There are several options available to the caregiver when they need more help either in the home or when making the decision to seek help on a regular (day care), temporary, respite, or permanent basis. Recognize your limitations and seek help. It is important that you make this decision at the appropriate time for you. The statistics are quite clear: Due to the stress of caregiving, caregivers suffer greater rates of depression, comorbid illnesses, and face death, on average, 15 years sooner than those without caregiver responsibilities.

Home Care
Visiting nurses, home health aides, homemakers, and paid companions can provide services at home such as bathing, dressing, providing meals, or companionship while you take a break. The family usually pays for these services that can be provided by Home Health Agencies found in the yellow pages or on the Home Health Care website for your state. Make sure that the agency you choose has staff trained in Alzheimer's disease care and they are able to provide trained staff to you. Consider a combination of in-home care with social model day care, as this will benefit the person with Alzheimer's. In some states, these agencies are not licensed. If so, you can consider residential care as an alternative. Consider the costs carefully. In-home care is generally more expensive than residential care/assisted living and is often as costly as skilled nursing. Home care may not be the best option for someone if social model day care is not involved on a daily basis. Home care sends one caregiver that may or may not be trained in dementia/Alzheimer's care. This can cause significant behavioral issues for the person with Alzheimer's, as the caregiver may not understand redirection/validation or how to communicate with someone who has Alzheimer's. As well, the individual may not thrive under home care alone as there is a lack of social interaction. Just you and a caregiver are not sufficient interaction. The person needs more than you can provide to help keep them active and challenged.

Respite/Short-Term Residential Care
Residential facilities offer short-term stays from a few days to a few weeks to give caregivers a chance to take a break.

Day Care

This option is used for the patient who is in the mild to moderate and moderate to severe stages of Alzheimer's disease as long as they can still benefit from socialization and activities. This setting encourages independence, decision making in a protective environment, and the use of remaining cognitive abilities. In turn, this type of participation enhances self-esteem, self-respect, the sense of belonging, the feeling of accomplishment, and the sense of purpose.

The caregiver also benefits from this arrangement by gaining some time to themselves, to relax or do things important to them. The working caregiver does not have to leave work and create a financial crisis, but is able to maintain an active work schedule knowing that the patient is in a safe environment. The caregiver spouse has the opportunity to be free of worry, fulfill personal needs, work, or visit friends. When the patient returns home, the family members are more ready to deal with the situation and the patient has had a fulfilling day, is content, less frustrated, and ready to be with the family. Some day care centers cost nothing, some are on a sliding scale, and some have a set fee. The number of days attending is optional, but it is advisable to use a minimum of 2 set days a week to establish routine. Select your times based on space availability, but a minimum of 2 days a week is needed to benefit the individual. All residents require a current tuberculosis (TB) test prior to enrollment.

Assisted Living Facilities

An assisted living facility or residential care community is a long-term care alternative, licensed by the state. It may be a private home or large, apartment-like facility that provides personal services to the residents. These services include assistance with eating, bathing, grooming, dressing, walking, housekeeping, supervision of self-administered medication, and arrangement for or provision of social and leisure services. The staff does not provide dental, medical, nursing, or mental health services. This arrangement is appropriate for the Alzheimer's disease patient as long as skilled care is not required due to severe decline in capabilities, impaired ambulation, severe behaviors, or additional medical problems. Assisted living facilities are paid for by family members or some long-term care insurance. They are generally one-third to one-half of the cost of nursing homes.

Assisted living facilities often have small units for dementia/Alzheimer's. Look into their community's design, resident policies, training, and behavior management strategies. Consider facilities that offer the social model program where there are large outdoor areas that residents can freely access, nursing staff, a medical director specialized in Alzheimer's, and a staff training program for Alzheimer's. The social model program supports the cognitive and social needs of those with Alzheimer's. Good programs will go on throughout the day and will be appropriate for adults.

Nursing Home Care
Nursing homes provide total care and are appropriate for those patients in the later stages of Alzheimer's disease. This service may be paid for in the following ways:

o Private pay.
o Medicare — Only up to 100 days after 3-day hospital stay for treatable problem. Does not cover custodial care (which is what Alzheimer's patients require).
o Medicaid — If patient and spouse qualify medically and financially, may pay some of the cost through Institutional Care Program.
o VA benefits — If patient qualifies.
o Long-term care insurance — If policy was in effect prior to the diagnosis of the disease.

Hospice
Hospice is for the terminally ill person with Alzheimer's disease and is focused on late-stage care and end-of-life decisions. End-of-life decisions should respect the patient's values and wishes and maintain their comfort and dignity. If there are no advance directives in place, a family must be prepared to make decisions consistent with what they believe the person's wishes would have been in combination with their best interests. If advance directives are in place, make sure that others know about them and are involved in the medical decision-making process. Give documents

to family and health care providers and make sure that they are placed in the medical record. Do not assume family, doctors, or other health care providers understand the directives. Talk to them and be involved in working out the health care plan based on the advance directives.

Internet Resources:
There are numerous Internet sites that offer information that may be of use to you. We do not endorse any but here are a few that were still operational when we went to press.

www.assistedlivinginfo.com/
www.seniorlivingonline.com/
www.newlifestyles.com/
http://seniorliving.about.com/od/housingoptions/
www.caregiver.org
www.aoa.gov/prof/aoaprog/caregiver/caregiver.asp

8. Support

It is essential for your well being that you put together a support group to help you when taking care of your patient as well as to provide support for yourself. Support will take different forms depending on your needs at any given time, but certainly you should expect that the need for support will increase with time. Support may come from family and friends; governmental, informal, and specialized organizations; religious groups; and from information sources such as the Internet. It is never too early to start thinking about putting together your support group once you know that you will be the caregiver.

Find out which of your family members and friends you can rely on to help you with various tasks, transportation, moral support, conversation partner, etc. Also, make up your own mind as to what degree you think you will be able to rely on them. Some people are simply unreliable — they say the right things and they mean well, but when it comes to crunch time, they are nowhere to be found. These are people you may choose to keep as friends, for conversation, or for a cup of coffee, but you do not want to be in a position of having them let you down when you really need their help and their presence. Pick out the family members and friends you can count on and talk to them about what you might want them to do. Make sure that they understand the level of support you are expecting from them. Give them the chance to tell you what they can and cannot do, or what they are prepared to do. Keep in mind that you are going to need people that live close by. Also, they have their own lives to lead and their responsibilities to their own families, and there will be times when they will have higher priorities and will not be able to do what you expect. For this reason, you should have as wide a support group as possible to make sure that you have backup when you need it.

In addition to support from family and friends, there are more formal support groups that are there to help you when you need advice based on experience with the Alzheimer's patient. These support groups are often available in your community and they may provide free or low-cost services such as transportation or meals delivered to the home. Make a point to find out what community resources are available in your area. The Alzheimer's Association is an excellent starting point to find out what is available for you locally. If you are a member of a religious organization, they are often able to help either by providing services or advising you of what services are available in your community.

The organized support groups can provide many benefits, such as providing a forum where you can talk to others. Sharing experiences with those in a similar situation can be helpful when dealing with the stress of caregiving and provides an opportunity to:

- o Meet new friends and acquaintances.
- o Learn from others and share with others
    - Experiences with Alzheimer's
    - Available resources in your community.
- o Express your negative feelings in an environment where you are understood and not criticized.
- o Receive moral support and encouragement and feel better about yourself.
- o Get out of the house.

There is a great deal of information available on the Internet. We have provided some URLs below to help you find the information that you will need. Chat rooms on the Internet can provide a source of information, the opportunity to share experiences, and obtain useful advice from other caregivers, but a word of caution is needed before you heed the advice of unqualified people: Check with your doctor before making any changes to the plan of care or to the daily routine. However, information alone will not be enough; you will need human support from your family and friends and from the organized support groups.

Internet Resources
By no means exhaustive, this list of contact websites will help you to find more information on Alzheimer's disease and the resources that are available to you. If you have time to browse the Internet,

simply typing "Alzheimer's disease" into your favorite search engine will provide you with a wealth of information.

Alzheimer's Disease International — www.alz.co.uk
The Alzheimer's Association (USA) — www.alz.org
Alzheimer's Foundation of America – www.alzfdn.org
Alzheimer's Disease Education and Referral Center — www.alzheimers.org
Children of Aging Parents — www.caps4caregivers.org
Eldercare Locator — www.eldercare.gov
Family Caregiver Alliance — www.caregiver.org
National Institute on Aging — www.nia.nih.gov
Medline Plus — Alzheimer's disease
www.nlm.nih.gov/medlineplus/alzheimersdisease.html
Alzheimer's Family Relief Program (financial assistance) — www.ahaf.org/afrp/afrp.htm
alzinfo.org — www.alzinfo.org/community/
National Healthy Aging Campaign -www.healthyaging.net

A list of Alzheimer's chat rooms can be found at: www.chatmag.com/topics/health/alzheimers.html

9. Scientific and Medical Basis of Alzheimer's Disease

Najeeb Qadi, MD and Sandra Tam, MSc
Department of Medicine (Neurology), University of British Columbia

Correspondence to: Sandra Tam, Division of Neurology, Vancouver Hospital and Health Sciences Center S192, 2211 Wesbrook Mall, Vancouver, BC V6T 2B5. E-mail: sandra.tam@telus.net

Alzheimer's Disease and the Brain

Dementia is a condition where a person has a progressive loss of intellectual functions (such as thinking, memory, reasoning, and language) to such an extent that it interferes with daily functioning. There are many causes of dementia, with Alzheimer's disease being the leading cause. Alzheimer's has been estimated to affect 6–7% of the population over the age of 65, increasing by twofold every 5 years[1]. An individual with this disease has trouble remembering, speaking, learning, making judgments, and planning. Some people feel restless and moody. It may take many years for Alzheimer's to express itself.

There are very important changes that occur in the brain in Alzheimer's. To understand these changes, it helps to understand how the brain functions.

The brain has millions of nerve cells called neurons that carry information in the form of electrical impulses. The electrical charge causes neurons to release chemicals (neurotransmitters) that move between nerve cells across a small gap (synapse). This is illustrated in Figure 1. These messages allow the brain to think, remember, and direct our body movement.

The cerebrum makes up the largest section of the brain. Its surface has many deep fissures (sulci) and convolutions (gyri), giving it a wrinkled appearance. It has two halves (hemispheres) that are

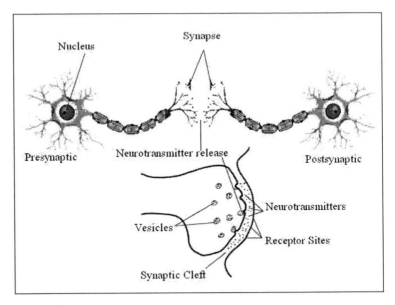

Figure 1: Neuron

connected by a thick band of nerve fibers. As seen in Figure 2, each half of the cerebrum is made up of four lobes:

1   The occipital lobe, located in the back of the brain, handles visual information.

2   The parietal lobe, lying above the occipital lobe, plays an important role in sorting and interpreting information from the various senses.

3   In the front of the brain is the frontal lobe. This lobe has functions that include cognitive (complex thinking, language, reasoning, problem solving) and behavioral features (impulse control, judgment, sexual behavior, socialization).

4   The temporal lobe is located beneath the frontal lobe. This lobe functions in hearing, language, and speech, as well as in memory. There is a very important structure on the inside of the temporal lobe, the hippocampus, which is essential for short-term memory.

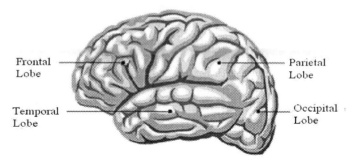

| Frontal Lobe | | Parietal Lobe |
| Temporal Lobe | | Occipital Lobe |

Figure 2: Cerebrum

Neurotransmitters
Neurotransmitters are the chemicals that neurons use to transmit messages to one another and to the rest of the body. After the chemicals are released from the neurons, they travel across the synapses and bind to receptors on nearby cells. There are several types of neurotransmitters in the brain, each has differing functions. Some are excitatory (causing nerve stimulation), whereas others are inhibitory (inhibiting nerve stimulation).

Glutamate is the most common excitatory neurotransmitter in the brain. Studies have identified glutamate as being critical in the formation of memory as well as the generation of new connections between neurons. Glutamate triggers the receptors on a target nerve cell, called N-methyl-D-aspartate (NMDA) receptors, to allow the right amount of calcium to flow in the nerve cell. This is necessary for nerve cells to function normally and, in particular, to store information[2]. Without enough glutamate, the chemical environment for successful transmission and formation of memory is not created. Information cannot be stored. On the other hand, too much glutamate or calcium can damage nerve cells[3].

Acetylcholine is another type of excitatory neurotransmitter. It functions both within the brain and throughout the body. In the brain, it is important in cognition and memory. In the body, it controls salivation, heart rate, sweating, and muscle movements.

Acetylcholine is quickly removed from the synapse by a special enzyme called acetylcholinesterase that breaks it down to its original chemical components. These components are not active and are then recycled to make more acetylcholine. Another enzyme like acetylcholinesterase is called butyrylcholinesterase. This enzyme also aids in the breakdown of acetylcholine.

As you can see, the brain is a complex organ indeed!

Pathophysiology of Alzheimer's Disease
In individuals with Alzheimer's disease, the cerebrum undergoes a degenerative process. This means that nerve cells age and die prematurely. In turn, the volume of the brain shrinks. This difference of the cerebrum between a normal brain and one with Alzheimer's is seen in Figure 3.

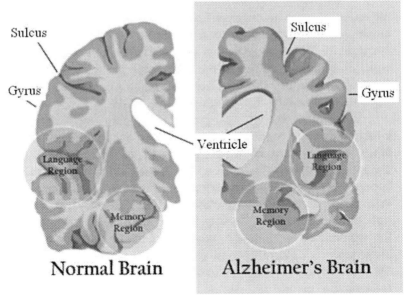

Figure 3: Coronal section of a normal brain vs. Alzheimer's brain

We now understand that there are some characteristic footprints of Alzheimer's. The formation of amyloid plaques and neurofibrillary tangles, as seen in Figure 4, are invariable findings in Alzheimer's.

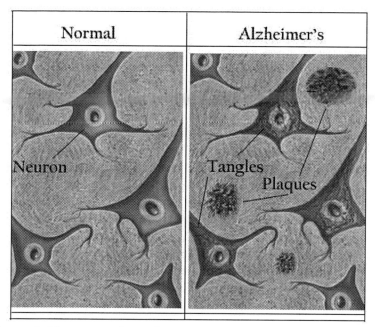

Figure 4: Plaques and tangles

Plaques and tangles are protein deposits that form in or near neurons. Though it is normal for some of these deposits to form as we age, an excessive number of these occur in Alzheimer's.[4,5].

The protein that makes up plaques is found as a natural constituent in the body. This protein is called amyloid. Plaques are abnormal, sticky clusters of amyloid. They are found in the spaces between the neurons and can disrupt the pathways that carry signals from one neuron to the other.

Tangles are made up of a protein called tau that is also found naturally in the body. In Alzheimer's, the protein gets "tangled" up. Tangles look like threads twisted around each other and are found inside the neurons. Tangles prevent neurons from functioning normally. Some researchers believe that tangles seriously damage the neurons, leading to their death.

When neurons are clogged with tangles and the spaces between neurons are clogged with plaques, the transmission of nerve impulses from one neuron to the next does not happen properly. As a result, the brain has difficulty performing mental functions, such as remembering and thinking.

One of the most important symptoms of Alzheimer's is memory loss. This occurs because plaques and tangles deposit in the memory centers of the brain very early. This can be seen from neuroimaging testing with CT or MRI. The entorhinal cortex (the gateway for information leading to the hippocampus) and the hippocampus are among the first regions to be affected[6,7]. This is caused by the death of up to 50% of the neurons in those areas. Another region of the brain that shows significant neuronal death is the nucleus basalis, which contains many neurons that use acetylcholine as chemical messengers[8,9,10]. Damage to this region reduces the transmission of messages along the pathways using acetylcholine.

As Alzheimer's progresses, these brain changes become more widespread until, eventually, the whole brain is affected.

The current therapies are mainly targeted at neurotransmitter problems in Alzheimer's. There is a group of acetylcholinesterase inhibitors (Donepezil, Rivastigmine, and Galantamine) that help to reduce the symptoms by blocking the breakdown of acetylcholine and improving neuronal communication. Butyrylcholinesterase inhibitors can also act in a similar way. The NMDA receptors antagonist (Memantine) blocks glutamate from binding to its receptor on the nerve cell. This action is associated with some improvement in Alzheimer's symptoms.

To date, we do not fully understand the causes of Alzheimer's. We do realize, however, that a complex series of changes occur in the brain over a long period of time. As these changes spread throughout the brain, the disease becomes increasingly severe. Researchers are attempting to elucidate the processes that trigger and promote these changes. As our knowledge increases, so will our ability to find suitable treatments that may in time lead to the cure of this disease.

125

Acknowledgment
The authors gratefully acknowledge Dr. Howard Feldman for his expertise and assistance in preparing this article.

References

1 Canadian Study of Health and Aging: Study methods and prevalence of dementia. Canadian Study of Health and Aging Working Group. CMAJ 1994, 150:899–912.

2 Shimizu E, Tang YP, Rampon C, Tsien JZ: NMDA receptor-dependent synaptic reinforcement is a crucial process for memory consolidation. Science 2000, 290:1170–1174.

3 Lipton SA, Rosenberg PA: Excitatory amino acids as a final common pathway for neurologic disorders. N Engl J Med 1994, 330:613–622.

4 Khachaturian ZS: Diagnosis of Alzheimer's disease. Arch Neurol 1985, 42(11):1097–1105.

5 Mirra SS, Heyman A, McKeel D, Sumi SM, Crain BJ, Brownlee LM, Vogel FS, Hughes JP, van Belle G, Berg L: The Consortium to Establish a Registry for Alzheimer's Disease (CERAD). Part II. Standardization of the neuropathologic assessment of Alzheimer's disease. Neurology 1991, 41(4):479–486.

6 Price JL, Ko AI, Wade MJ, Tsou SK, McKeel DW, Morris JC: Neuron number in the entorhinal cortex and CA1 in preclinical Alzheimer disease. Arch Neurol 2001, 58(9):1395–1402.

7 Killiany RJ, Hyman BT, Gomez-Isla T, Moss MB, Kikinis R, Jolesz F, Tanzi R, Jones K, Albert MS: MRI measures of entorhinal cortex vs hippocampus in preclinical AD. Neurology 2002, 58(8):1188–1196.

8 Whitehouse PJ, Price DL, Struble RG, et al.: Alzheimer's disease and senile dementia: loss of neurons in the basal forebrain. Science 1982, 215:1237–1239.

9 Bartus RT, Dean RL, Beer B, et al.: The cholinergic hypothesis of geriatric memory dysfunction. Science 1982, 217:408–417.

10 Coyle JT, Price DL, DeLong MR: Alzheimer's disease: a disorder of central cholinergic innervation. Science 1983, 219:1184–1190.

126

Further Reading

Afifi A, Bergman R: Functional Neuroanatomy: Text and Atlas. 1st edition, New York: McGraw-Hill, 1998.

Cummings JL: Alzheimer's disease. N Engl J Med 2004, 351:56–67.

Fix J: High-Yield Neuroanatomy. 3rd edition. Philadelphia/Baltimore: Lippincott Williams & Wilkins, 2002.

Fonnum F: Glutamate: a neurotransmitter in mammalian brain. J Neurochem 1984, 42:1–11.

Gauthier S: Clinical Diagnosis and Management of Alzheimer's Disease. 2nd edition, London: Martin Dunitz, Nov 2000.

McDonald WM, Nemeroff CB: Neurotransmitters and neuropeptides in Alzheimer's disease. Psychiatr Clin North Am 1991, 14(2):421–442.

Mendez M, Cummings J: Dementia: A Clinical Approach. 3rd edition, Oxford: Butterworth-Heinemann, July 2003.

Orrego F, Villanueva S: The chemical nature of the main central excitatory transmitter: a critical appraisal based upon release studies and synaptic vesicle localization. Neuroscience 1993, 56:539–555.

Introduction to Genetics and Alzheimer's Disease
Jeffrey Hillier PhD

A genetic cause for Alzheimer's disease is indicated both in those patients who have family members with the disease and in Alzheimer's disease without any family history of the disease. The term Familial Alzheimer's Disease (FAD) is used when two or more members of a family have Alzheimer's. FAD represents about 25% of all Alzheimer's cases and is diagnosed as early-onset (<2%) when onset occurs between ages 30 and 65, and late-onset (~23%) when onset occurs after age 65.

Many of our readers will be aware that chromosomes contain DNA, a large double stranded molecule (double helix) that includes genes, and functions in the transmission of hereditary information. Humans have 23 pairs of chromosomes, designated 1 to 22 in order of decreasing size with the 23rd chromosome being the sex chromosome designated X and Y for the female and male respectively.

The genes are the basic physical units of heredity that provide the coded instructions for synthesis of RNA, which, when transcribed into protein, leads to the expression of hereditary character. When genetic mutations occur or when genes are damaged, this process whereby DNA makes RNA makes proteins is disrupted and incorrect proteins are made. These incorrect proteins can, in some cases, be the cause of disease.

One of the proteins commonly found in our blood as a carrier of cholesterol is called apolipoprotein E (apoE). The apoE gene that produces apolipoprotein E is found on Chromosome 19 and has been found to be common to many family members who have developed Alzheimer's disease and is linked to the most common form of Alzheimer's, late-onset Alzheimer's disease. Apolipoprotein E is much more common among Alzheimer's patients than in the general population.

The gene that produces apolipoprotein E is found in several different forms called alleles. There are three alleles named apoE2, apoE3 and apoE4. Of these three alleles apoE3 is the most common while apoE4 is found in about forty percent of late onset Alzheimer's patients compared to its existence in about 15% of the general population. ApoE4 is found both in Alzheimer's patients who have a family history of Alzheimer's disease and in patients with no known family history. The apoE4 gene appears to be associated with the risk for developing Alzheimer's disease. People with the apoE3 gene have less risk than those carrying the apoE4 gene. People carrying the apoE2 gene have the least risk of developing Alzheimer's. If you inherit the apoE4 gene from both your father and your mother you are eight times more likely to develop Alzheimer's disease than if you inherit the apoE3 gene from both parents.

So why is this? It turns out that the apoE4 protein (transcribed from the apoE4 gene) binds rapidly and tightly to β amyloid while the apoE3 protein does not. Normally in the human body β amyloid is soluble, but when it binds with the apoE4 protein β amyloid becomes insoluble making it possible for it to be deposited in plaques; the kind of plaques seen in the brains of Alzheimer's patients.

Further links between the apoE4 protein and Alzheimer's disease have been suggested based on research studies. The protein tau exists normally in the human body and is a primary component of neuronal microtubules that are involved in regulating the structure and assembly of the neuron. The apoE4 protein causes the structure to somehow unravel and produce the kind of neurofibrillary tangles found in the brains of patients with Alzheimer's disease. Another observation is that apoE4 has been associated with neurons with shorter dendrites limiting the communication with other neurons. This dendritic pruning also occurs in people without the apoE4 allele, but it happens twenty to thirty years later.

Other gene mutations have been identified in patients with early-onset familial Alzheimer's disease (FAD). A mutation on a gene on chromosome 21 is common and also a gene on chromosome 14.

The National Institute on Aging has launched a new effort to identify the genes that play a role in the development of Alzheimer's disease. They are seeking families with a family history of Alzheimer's disease to participate in the study. For details see http://ncrad.iu.edu/.

Glossary

Acetylcholine (ACh) — A neurotransmitter, the levels of which are significantly lowered in the brain with Alzheimer's disease.

Acetylcholinesterase (AChE) — An enzyme whose function is to break down acetylcholine so that it becomes ineffective as a neurotransmitter. Conversely, when this enzyme is inhibited (see acetylcholinesterase inhibitors), the efficacy of acetylcholine is enhanced.

Acetycholinesterase Inhibitors — A class of drugs whose function is to inhibit the activity of acetylcholinesterase and so enhance the efficacy of acetylcholine as a neurotransmitter.

Activities of Daily Living (ADLs) — ADLs are compromised in the Alzheimer's patient.

Advance Directive — A legal document that indicates the type of medical care a person wants to receive once they can no longer make or express these decisions due to incapacity. Two common forms of advance directive are Living Will and Durable Power of Attorney for Health Care.

Agnosia — Failure to recognize or identify objects despite intact sensory function.

Allele — any one of the alternate forms of a gene that occupy a specific position on a specific chromosome. Usually arising through mutation, alleles are responsible for hereditary variation.

Anomia — The inability to find the right word for an object.

Antipsychotics — A class of drugs that alleviate the symptoms of psychotic behaviors such as schizophrenia.

Aphasia — Language disturbance.

Apraxia — Impaired ability to carry out motor activities despite intact motor function.

Aricept (Donepezil HCl) — An anticholinesterase inhibitor that has been shown to be effective in slowing the progression of Alzheimer's in mild to moderate cases.

Assisted Living Facility — For people needing assistance with activities of daily living (ADLs), but wishing to live as independently as possible for as long as possible. Assisted living exists to bridge the gap between independent living and nursing homes.

Atrophy — Decrease in size or wasting away of a body part or tissue.

Biochemical Marker — Used to track the course of the disease and may provide a diagnostic test for the disease. A biochemical compound is identified whose concentrations change in relation to a critical pathogenic feature of the disease. For biochemical markers to be useful in everyday clinical situations, it is essential that the sensitivity and specificity are the same early on in the course of Alzheimer's and later in disease progression.

BMI — Body mass index.

Butyrylcholinesterase (BuChE) — An enzyme found in human brain neurons, glia, and in high levels in the plaques and tangles of Alzheimer's patients. The activity of BuChE in the brain increases with age (>60 years) and is raised in Alzheimer's patients.

Butyrylcholinesterase Inhibitors — A class of drugs that inhibits butyrylcholinesterase in the brain and may provide benefit to mild to moderate Alzheimer's patients.

Catastrophic Reaction — Disproportionate response due to a person's inability to handle multiple stimuli.

Cerebrospinal Fluid (CSF) — A fluid found in the brain and spinal cord that serves to maintain a uniform pressure within the central nervous system (CNS).

Cholinesterase Inhibitors — See acetylcholinesterase inhibitors and butyrylcholinesterase inhibitors.

Chromosome — A strand of DNA and associated proteins in the nucleus of eukaryotic cells that carries the genes and functions in the transmission of hereditary information. Humans have 23 pairs, designated 1 to 22 in order of decreasing size and X and Y for the female and male sex chromosomes respectively.

Cognex (Tacrine HCl) — A cholinesterase inhibitor that has been found to be useful in slowing the progression of the disease in Alzheimer's patients with mild to moderate symptoms.

Cognitive Baseline Evaluation — An initial evaluation of cognitive function that serves as a baseline for comparing progress associated with the interventions or progression of the disease.

Cognitive Impairment, Not Dementia (CIND) — See Mild Cognitive Impairment (MCI).

Combination Therapy — Two or more drugs when used in combination have a more beneficial effect than either drug alone.

Comorbidity — Pathological or disease conditions that are unrelated to the primary disease (Alzheimer's in this case), but occur at the same time.

Computed Tomography (CT) — A method of examining body organs by scanning them with X-rays and using a computer to construct a series of cross-sectional scans along a single axis.

Cortex — The outer layer of gray matter (unmyelinated neurons) that covers the cerebral hemispheres of the brain.

CPR — Cardiopulmonary resuscitation.

Dementia — Deterioration of intellectual faculties, such as memory, concentration, and judgment resulting from an organic disease or a disorder of the brain. It is sometimes accompanied by emotional disturbance and personality changes.

Dementia Risk Score — A new risk factor analysis used to try to predict which people may develop dementia.

DNA (deoxyribonucleic acid) — a polynucleotide that is the main component of chromosomes and is the material that carries the genetic information in the cell and is capable of self replication and the synthesis of RNA. DNA consists of two long chains of nucleotides twisted into a double helix and joined by hydrogen bonds between the complementary bases adenine and thymine or cytosine and guanine. The sequence of nucleotides determines individual hereditary characteristics.

DNR — Do not resuscitate.

Durable Power of Attorney for Health Care — A document that allows the patient to appoint a person (spouse, trusted family member, or friend) to make decisions about the patient's care and treatment. See also, Medical Power of Attorney and Health Care Surrogate.

Dysarthria — Poorly articulated speech.

Early-onset — In Alzheimer's disease patients, refers to the onset of the disease before the age of 65.

Echolalia — Repetition of someone's words over and over, as if echoing them.

Electroencephalography (EEG) — A method of recording the electrical activity of the brain using an electroencephalograph.

Executive Function — Abstract thinking.

Exelon (Rivastigmine HCl) — A cholinesterase inhibitor that has been found to be useful in slowing the progression of the disease in Alzheimer's patients with mild to moderate symptoms.

Familial — in Alzheimer's disease refers to the occurrence of two or more family members with Alzheimer's disease.

FAQ — Functional activities questionnaire.

FTD — Frontotemporal dementia. See page 28.

Gene — the basic physical unit of heredity; a linear sequence of nucleotides along a segment of DNA that provides the coded instructions for synthesis of RNA, which, when translated into protein, leads to the expression of hereditary character.

Gene Therapy — The insertion of genetically altered genes into cells to replace defective genes or to provide a specific disease-fighting function.

HAI — Hypoxic-anoxic injury of the brain.

Hallucination — The visual perception of an object that is not present.

Health Care Surrogate — A person appointed to make health care decisions for the patient when they become unable to make such decisions for themselves. The patient has no say in who becomes their health care surrogate. The patient can avoid having a health care surrogate appointed by appointing a medical power of attorney while they are able. See also, Medical Power of Attorney.

Hippocampus — A ridge in the floor of each lateral ventricle of the brain that consists mainly of gray matter and has a central role in memory processes. A part of the limbic system.

Hospice — A program that provides palliative care and attends to the emotional and spiritual needs of terminally ill patients at an inpatient facility or at the patient's home.

Late-onset — In Alzheimer's disease patients, refers to the onset of the disease after the age of 65.

Living Will — Written instructions that state the individual's preferences about the kinds of life-sustaining treatments they would or would not want to have and which should be withdrawn or withheld if the patient is terminally ill or facing imminent death.

LLD — Late-life depression.

Logoconia — Language difficulty in which the person repeats the first syllable of a word.

Magnetic Resonance Imaging (MRI) — The use of a nuclear magnetic resonance spectrometer to produce electronic images of specific atoms and molecular structures in solids, especially human cells, tissues, and organs.

Medicaid — A program providing medical care for the needy under joint federal and state participation in the U.S.

Medical Power of Attorney — A person appointed to make health care decisions for the patient after they become unable to make such decisions for themselves. They can specify what health care decisions their medical power of attorney can make.

Medicare — A federally sponsored health insurance and medical program for persons 65 and older in the U.S.

Medigap — Private health insurance designed to supplement the coverage provided under governmental programs such as Medicare in the U.S.

Memantine (Namenda) — The first and only representative of the class of drugs called NMDA receptor antagonists. Memantine has been shown to slow the progression of Alzheimer's in moderate to severe cases.

Memory (Immediate) — Type of memory in which information is remembered for only a few seconds.

Memory (Long-Term) — Memory that involves the storage and recall of information over a long period of time (as days, weeks, or years).

Memory (Remote) — Memory for things that happened in the distant past that are remembered long term.

Memory (Short-Term) — Memory that involves recall of information for a relatively short time (a few minutes or hours).

Mild Cognitive Impairment (MCI) — A classification of dementia that falls between normal memory loss from aging and Alzheimer's. Patients diagnosed with MCI are at a higher risk for developing Alzheimer's.

Mini Mental State Exam (MMSE) — A test of cognitive functions used to assist in the diagnosis of Alzheimer's. The test may be repeated during the progression of the disease as a measure of decline in cognitive function.

MRI — See magnetic resonance imaging.

Myoclonus – A sudden, irregular twitching of muscle resulting from a functional disorder of controlling motoneurons that occurs in various brain disorders.

Neuritic Plaques — Abnormal deposits of amyloid protein found in brain tissue lesions of people with Alzheimer's and other neurodegenerative diseases. Typically found coexisting with neurofibrillary tangles in Alzheimer's.

Neurofibrillary Tangles — Abnormal twisted bundles of neurofibrils found in brain tissue lesions of people with Alzheimer's and other neurodegenerative diseases. Typically found coexisting with neuritic plaques in Alzheimer's disease..

Neuroleptic — A tranquilizing drug, especially one used in treating mental disorders.

Neuron — A cell that is specialized to conduct nerve impulses in the central nervous system and the peripheral nervous system.

Neurotransmitter — Any of the various chemical substances, such as acetylcholine, glutamate, norepinephrine, serotonin that transmit nerve impulses across a synapse.

NMDA — N-methyl-D-aspartate.

NMDA Receptor Antagonists — A class of drugs (Memantine is currently the only one approved for the treatment of Alzheimer's) that work by blocking the NMDA receptor at nerve synapses.

NPH — Normal pressure hydrocephalus.

NSAIDs — Nonsteroidal anti-inflammatory drugs.

Nursing Home — A private establishment that provides living quarters and care for the elderly or the chronically ill.

Palilalia — Repetition of a particular word.

Pathophysiology — The functional changes or the study of such changes associated with or resulting from disease or injury.

Positron Emission Tomography (PET) — Tomography in which a computer-generated image of a biological activity within the body is produced through the detection of gamma rays that are emitted when introduced radionuclides decay and release positrons.

Physical Self-Maintenance Scale (PSMS) — Tests the patient's ability to perform basic self-maintenance tasks such as using the toilet, eating, dressing, grooming, bathing, and getting around. The test is given by the caregiver or the doctor during diagnosis and again several times during the course of the disease to monitor change. The patient's scores will increase as the disease progresses.

Power of Attorney (POA) — A legal document that gives another person the authority to manage the patient's property.

Prion — A protein particle, lacking nucleic acid, thought to be implicated in causing various neurodegenerative diseases such as Creutzfeldt-Jacob disease, scrapie, and bovine spongiform encephalopathy (mad cow disease).

Protein — Proteins are fundamental components of all living cells and include many substances, such as enzymes, hormones, and antibodies, that are necessary for the proper functioning of an organism.

PSP — Progressive Supranuclear Palsy.

Psychotropic — Exerting an effect on the mind or mental capacities.

Reminyl (Galantamine HBr) — A cholinesterase inhibitor that has been found to be useful in slowing the progression of the disease in Alzheimer's patients with mild to moderate symptoms.

Respite Care — Provides short-term, full-time care for patients in order to give the caregiver a respite.

RNA (ribonucleic acid) — a polymeric constituent of all living cells and many viruses transcribed from DNA in the cell nucleus or in the mitochondrion or chloroplast (in plants), containing along the strand a linear sequence of nucleotide bases that is complementary to the DNA strand from which it is transcribed: the composition of the RNA molecule is identical with that of DNA except for the substitution of the sugar ribose for deoxyribose and the substitution of the nucleotide base uracil for thymine. The structure and base sequence of RNA are determinants of protein synthesis and the transmission of genetic information.

Safe Return Program — A nationwide system designed to identify, locate, and return Alzheimer's sufferers who may wander from the home. For more information call 1-800-272-3900 or to register call 1-888-872-8566.

Single Photon Emission Computed Tomography (SPECT) — Similar to X-ray computed tomography (CT) or magnetic resonance imaging (MRI), SPECT allows us to visualize functional information about a patient's specific organ or body system. Internal radiation is administered by means of a pharmaceutical, which is labeled with a radioactive isotope. This so-called radiopharmaceutical, or tracer, is either injected, ingested, or inhaled. The radioactive isotope decays, resulting in the emission of gamma rays. These gamma rays give us a picture of what is happening inside the patient's body.

Social Model Day Care — A day care facility offering a program that focuses on quality of life for the resident. Social model programs are designed to help the cognitive, social, and physical needs of the person with Alzheimer's and concentrate on improving overall quality of life for the individual while giving sense of purpose and community.

Sundowner's Syndrome — People with Alzheimer's have more behavior problems in the evening or around "sundown." The frustrations and sensory stimulation build up throughout the day and, by "sundown," they are not able to cope as well with the confusing environment around them. They may become increasingly confused, agitated, and anxious and may pace the floor, begin to wander, or show other nervous behavior.

Synapse — The junction across which a nerve impulse passes from an axon terminal to a neuron, a muscle cell, or a gland cell. Nerve impulses cross a synapse through the action of neurotransmitters.

Tomography — Methods of obtaining pictures of the interior of the body.

UTI — Urinary tract infection.

Vascular Dementia — See page 29.